"Unbroken Harmony:

A Journey of Hope and Resilience"

Pre face

As I sit down to write this preface, I am struck by the journey that has led me to these pages. This book, while a work of fiction, is deeply rooted in the universal truths and struggles that many of us face. It is a story born from the heartaches, triumphs, and resilient spirits of countless individuals whom I have encountered, including myself, in the winding journey of life.

The seed for this book was planted during a particularly challenging phase of my life. As a single parent, I have navigated the turbulent waters of raising a child alone, all while trying to heal from the scars of past traumas. It is a path marked by immense challenges, yet also by incredible growth and unexpected joys. This story is a reflection of that journey – an amalgamation of the myriad experiences, emotions, and lessons learned along the way.

In writing this book, my hope is to reach out to those who may find themselves in the shoes of Anna, the protagonist of our story. Anna's experiences, though fictional, mirror the realities of many. Her journey is one of facing past demons, embracing the present, and courageously stepping into the future. It is a narrative of finding strength in vulnerability, hope in despair, and companionship in the most unlikely places.

This book is also a tribute to the silent warriors – the single parents who juggle the roles of nurturer, provider, and protector, all while bearing the weight of their personal battles. It is a recognition of their struggles, a celebration of their strength, and an acknowledgment of their unwavering love.

As you turn these pages, I invite you to journey with Anna. You may find pieces of your story reflected in hers. My deepest desire is that this story resonates with you, offering comfort, understanding, and perhaps a new perspective on your own journey.

Remember, in the grand tapestry of life, every struggle is significant, every challenge is a lesson, and every heartache carries the promise of growth and renewal. May you find in this story a reflection of your resilience, a whisper of hope, and a testament to the enduring strength of the human spirit.

With heartfelt sincerity,

Kyleen

Chapter 1:

"Shattered Dreams"

The first light of dawn crept gently into the room, its soft illumination revealing the modest surroundings of Anna's living space. The living room, small yet cozy, bore the marks of a life lived with simplicity and care. The walls were adorned with Lily's colorful drawings, each a masterpiece of a child's imagination, depicting suns with smiling faces and houses with crooked windows. A small, well-worn sofa sat against one wall; its cushions slightly sunken from years of use but still inviting.

In her bedroom, the quiet moments of early morning were a sanctuary for Anna, where her thoughts roamed freely in the solitude. The room, bathed in the soft hues of dawn, held a comforting familiarity. The ceiling above, an old friend, bore witness to her deepest thoughts and restless nights. Its surface, painted a gentle cream, was textured with subtle imperfections and the faint traces of a long-forgotten water stain, each blemish known by heart and woven into the tapestry of her life.

Anna lay in her bed, nestled under a quilted blanket that bore the softness of years of use. The bed itself, a sturdy wooden frame, was positioned against the main wall, flanked by a pair of well-worn nightstands. On one, a small lamp with a faded shade cast a warm, inviting glow, its light dimmed for the quiet hours of the morning.

The room was a reflection of Anna herself – unassuming yet filled with quiet strength. The walls, adorned with a few carefully chosen pieces of art, spoke of her love for simple, meaningful beauty. A small bookshelf, overflowing with books of all genres, stood in one corner, a testament to her love for literature and learning. A cozy reading chair, its fabric worn in places, sat beside a window that looked out to a modest garden, her haven of greenery and blooms.

As for Anna, in these moments of introspection, she appeared a figure of resilience and contemplation. Her hair, a soft cascade of chestnut brown, was tousled from sleep, framing a face marked with the subtle lines of life's experiences. Her eyes, thoughtful and deep, reflected the myriad roles she played – mother, provider, protector. In her simple night attire, she was every bit the embodiment of a woman who had weathered storms and savored joys, her appearance marked not by vanity but by the authenticity of her journey.

The room, with its mix of simplicity and warmth, was a mirror of Anna's inner world – a place of refuge and reflection, of quiet strength and enduring hope. In this familiar space, Anna found both the freedom to ponder her worries and the courage to face the day ahead, her mind weaving through the complexities of financial concerns, daily challenges, and the future she was building for herself and Lily.

Beside her, Lily, her daughter and the center of her world, slept peacefully. The soft moonlight filtering through the curtains cast a gentle glow on Lily's features, accentuating her youthful innocence. Lily, now blossoming into a young teenager, still retained traces of the child she once was. Her face, relaxed in sleep, bore the soft roundness of childhood, yet was beginning to show the early contours of adolescence.

Lily's hair, a cascade of light brown curls, spread across her pillow, framing her face like a halo. Her long eyelashes, dark against her fair skin, lay closed, veiling the bright, curious eyes that Anna knew so well – eyes that sparkled with intelligence and a hint of mischievousness when awake. A slight smile played on Lily's lips, hinting at the pleasant dreams that danced in her slumbering mind.

As Anna watched her, she couldn't help but notice the subtle changes that were slowly transforming Lily from a child into a young woman. Her features were becoming more defined, losing the cherubic softness of earlier years. Yet, in her sleep, Lily seemed to retreat into the simpler realm of childhood, a world that Anna cherished and sought to protect.

Anna's gaze lingered on Lily's face, taking in the gentle rise and fall of her chest as she breathed quietly. In these quiet moments, Anna's heart swelled with a profound mix of emotions. Love was there, a deep, unconditional love that anchored her entire being. Worry too, a natural concern of a mother watching her child navigate the tricky path to adulthood. And there was determination, a quiet resolve to guide, protect, and empower Lily as she grew.

In Lily's peaceful, sleeping form, Anna saw both the child she had nurtured and the young woman Lily was becoming. It was a bittersweet reminder of the passage of time, the inevitable transformation that life brings, and the preciousness of each moment they shared.

With the relentless beep of the alarm clock, the day officially began. Anna's morning routine was a well-rehearsed ritual. She moved quietly, mindful of not waking Lily, as she picked out clothes for the day. Each action, from folding the blankets to selecting a comfortable yet practical outfit, was done with a practiced efficiency borne out of necessity.

In the kitchen, the act of brewing coffee was almost ceremonial for Anna. As she measured the grounds and listened to the gentle gurgle of the machine, the rich, earthy aroma of the coffee began to fill the small space. This scent, comforting and familiar, provided a brief respite and a sensory indulgence in her otherwise straightforward existence. Standing there, with the warm mug in her hands, Anna often found herself pausing in these small, seemingly mundane moments, allowing herself a brief interlude of reflection before the day's responsibilities took hold. This daily ritual, simple yet profound, served as a gentle segue into the rhythm of the day, a moment of tranquility before the whirlwind of activities began.

She glanced at the array of Lily's drawings pinned to the fridge, each a colorful reminder of the joy and creativity that her daughter brought into her life. It was these small tokens, these simple joys, that fortified her on the more challenging days. With a deep breath and a final sip of her coffee, Anna steeled herself for the day ahead, ready to face the world with the quiet strength that had become her trademark.

At the breakfast table, the conversation between Anna and Lily was sparse, a noticeable contrast to the lively chatter that used to bubble up effortlessly in the mornings of years past. Anna, sensing the quietness that had crept into their interactions, attempted to infuse some of the old energy back into their routine. She asked Lily about her school projects, trying to ignite a spark of excitement by talking about subjects she knew Lily enjoyed.

"How's the science project coming along?" Anna asked with a smile, passing the jam across the table. Lily offered a brief update, but her responses were short, lacking the enthusiastic detail that used to accompany such discussions. Anna then shifted to asking about Lily's plans for the day, hoping to stir some of the youthful enthusiasm her daughter was known for. However, despite her best efforts, the conversation invariably drifted back to the practicalities of daily life – homework that needed finishing, chores to be done, and gentle reminders about Lily's after-school activities.

With each pragmatic exchange, a pang of familiar guilt tugged at Anna's heart. She longed to delve into deeper, more meaningful conversations with Lily, to reconnect in a way that transcended the routine logistics of their day-to-day lives. This guilt, a constant companion, stemmed from her role as a single parent juggling the dual demands of providing and nurturing, always wondering if she was doing enough.

As they finished their breakfast, Anna cleared the table, her mind already racing through the list of tasks awaiting her at the bookstore and the college. She glanced at Lily, who was gathering her school things, and felt a silent promise rise within her – to find more moments of connection, to bridge the growing quiet with the warmth and openness they once shared so effortlessly.

The morning routine in Anna's household was a well-rehearsed dance against the clock, a flurry of activity that began the moment the alarm clock heralded the start of a new day. In the soft light of early morning, Anna would gently wake Lily, coaxing her out of the warm embrace of her dreams. The sound of their feet padding across the hardwood floor marked the beginning of their daily ritual.

In the bathroom, the sounds of brushing teeth and the rhythmic swish of water were accompanied by Anna's gentle reminders to Lily to hurry along. The mirror would fog up from the warm water, and they would take turns wiping it down, catching glimpses of each other's sleepy reflections.

In Lily's room, the task of choosing an outfit often became a negotiation, balancing Lily's growing desire for self-expression with practical considerations like the weather and school activities. Anna would help Lily comb her hair, sometimes braiding it or pulling it back into a neat ponytail, a routine that had become a cherished moment of mother-daughter bonding.

amidst last-minute checks of school bags to ensure that homework and projects were packed. Anna would fill Lily's water bottle and occasionally slip a small treat into her lunchbox, a little surprise to brighten her daughter's day.

As they stepped out of the apartment and locked the door, Anna would mentally run through her checklist – keys, wallet, phone, and Lily's school essentials. They descended the stairs and joined the stream of neighbors embarking on their own morning journeys.

Outside, the world was already in motion. The streets were alive with the sounds of traffic and the footsteps of hurried commuters. People moved with purpose, their minds focused on the destinations that awaited them. Anna, holding Lily's hand, navigated through the bustling crowd, feeling a stark contrast between the intimacy of their morning routine and the impersonal rush of the city.

Walking amidst the crowd, Anna felt enveloped by a sense of isolation, a poignant reminder of the solitary nature of her journey as a single parent. Surrounded by strangers, each absorbed in their own concerns, Anna's own challenges seemed invisible, her internal world unnoticed in the vast tapestry of the city's life. It was a moment of introspection, a silent acknowledgment of her strength and resilience in the face of life's ceaseless pace.

The morning walk to school, though brief, had blossomed into an invaluable ritual for Anna and Lily, a cherished interlude in their otherwise hectic day. Each step they took together along the familiar route was an opportunity for connection, a precious thread that continued to weave their close bond tighter.

As Anna and Lily strolled down the tree-lined streets of their neighborhood, their morning walk was enlivened by the comfortable and familiar rhythm of their conversation. The trees, a mix of oaks and maples, stood tall and sturdy, their leaves rustling softly in the gentle morning breeze, creating a natural canopy overhead. This path, trodden countless times, held memories of their shared laughter and quiet talks, an integral part of their daily routine.

Lily's stories, told with the unbridled enthusiasm and vivid imagination typical of her young age, were like colorful threads weaving through the fabric of their walk. She spoke of her latest art project with fervor, describing how she had boldly mixed blues and reds to create vibrant purples, her small hands gesticulating excitedly as she painted the scene in the air between them. Her eyes sparkled with pride as she recounted the praise she had received from her teacher, a moment that had clearly filled her with a sense of achievement and joy.

The simplicity of her tales, like those of her recess adventures - games of tag and make-believe worlds conjured with friends - offered Anna a precious glimpse into the innocence and wonder of childhood. These stories, though simple, were windows into Lily's world, filled with the purity and straightforwardness that adulthood often leaves behind.

Their bond was evident not just in their conversations but also in their playful interactions. Occasionally, they would stop to admire a particularly beautiful flower or an interesting bug on the sidewalk. Anna, ever encouraging of Lily's curiosity, would kneel beside her daughter, sharing in her wonder. These moments often turned into impromptu games – guessing the names of flowers or imagining the destinations of hurried ants.

As they walked, sometimes their roles would reverse, and it would be Anna sharing stories of her own childhood, much to Lily's delight. These tales were a bridge between generations, drawing them closer. Lily would listen, wide-eyed, as Anna recounted her own school day adventures, drawing parallels between their experiences, despite the years that separated them.

Their walk to school was more than just a physical journey; it was a daily reaffirmation of their connection. In these precious minutes, as they navigated the familiar route, hand in hand, they shared not just stories but parts of themselves, strengthening the invisible thread that bound them together. As they approached the school gates, where they would part ways for the day, they did so with the knowledge that this special time was theirs – a simple yet profound ritual that defined the essence of their relationship.

Anna, for her part, was an attentive audience, her responses and questions nurturing the flow of conversation. She marveled at Lily's creative spirit and her candid view of the world, each word from Lily a reminder of the beautiful simplicity of childhood. These conversations were windows into Lily's inner world, precious insights that Anna treasured.

In these moments, as they navigated the sidewalks bustling with other parents and children, their bond was palpable. It was evident in the way Lily's face lit up as she spoke, secure in the knowledge that she had her mother's undivided attention. It was reflected in Anna's responses, full of encouragement and affection, affirming the trust and openness that defined their relationship.

Anna often found herself silently observing Lily, noting the way her hair caught the sunlight or how her small hand felt in hers - firm and trusting. These observations were bittersweet, tinged with the awareness of time's relentless march. Anna wished she could slow down the clock, to preserve these moments of innocence and joy, to shield Lily from the inevitable complexities and challenges of growing up.

But as they neared the school gates, where Lily would soon slip away into her own world of classrooms and playgrounds, Anna recognized the importance of these morning walks. They were more than just a physical journey; they were a reinforcement of their unbreakable bond, a daily recommitment to their journey together as mother and daughter. It was in these fleeting, everyday moments that the depth and strength of their connection were most vividly brought to life.

At the school gates, their daily ritual of goodbye was a brief but poignant moment. Lily's small hand slipped from Anna's, a symbol of her growing independence. As Lily ran off to join her friends, her laughter echoed in Anna's ears, a bittersweet melody that lingered long after she had disappeared into the school. Anna stood there for a moment, caught between the joy of seeing her daughter happy and the ache of letting her go.

Turning away from the school, Anna began her walk to the bookstore where she worked. Each step felt heavy with the reluctance of a mother parting from her child. The familiar route to work was a time for Anna to brace herself for the day ahead, to shift from the role of mother to that of an employee, a switch that she had mastered but never found easy. As the bookstore came into view, Anna took a deep breath, readying herself to don the mask of normalcy that her job required, leaving her worries about Lily and their life at the doorstep.

Anna's workplace, was a charming haven tucked in a quaint street, sandwiched lovingly between a bustling café and an old-fashioned stationery shop. Its vintage sign, with gold lettering on a dark wood background, swung gently in the morning breeze, as if beckoning passersby to step into a world of stories and imagination.

Inside, the store was a labyrinth of bookshelves, reaching from floor to ceiling, filled with volumes that whispered tales of far-off places, epic adventures, and profound wisdom. The air was heavy with the scent of old paper and ink, a distinctive aroma that Anna had come to associate with comfort and escape. It was a sensory embrace, welcoming her into its fold each day.

Mark, her colleague, was already at the counter, arranging the display of new arrivals with meticulous care. His passion for books was evident in the way he handled each volume, as if they were precious treasures. His greeting to Anna was warm and genuine, a simple nod and smile that acknowledged their shared sanctuary in this haven of books. as Anna moved between the shelves, her mind inevitably wandered to chapters of her own life that she often wished she could rewrite. Her past relationship, a significant and tumultuous part of her history, often resurfaced in these solitary moments, bringing with it a tide of emotions.

Anna had once been in a relationship with someone she had deeply loved and trusted. This person, whom we'll call Ethan, had been a charming and seemingly caring partner at the start. They met during a period when Anna was discovering her own path, and Ethan's confident demeanor and promises of a future together had been intoxicating to her.

However, as time passed, the relationship began to reveal its darker facets. Ethan's charm gave way to control and manipulation. His words, which had once been filled with affection, turned sharp and critical. Anna found herself frequently on the receiving end of harsh criticisms and belittling comments, often about her aspirations and choices. Ethan's once-endearing attentiveness transformed into possessiveness, eroding Anna's sense of independence.

The relationship became a cycle of highs and lows, with moments of affection overshadowed by intense arguments and painful silences. Ethan's ability to oscillate between warmth and coldness left Anna in a state of constant emotional turmoil. The love she had felt turned into a source of confusion and pain.

The betrayal that ultimately ended their relationship wasn't just about infidelity; it was a betrayal of trust and the shared dreams they had built. When the truth came to light about Ethan's unfaithfulness, it was more than just a revelation of his actions. It represented the shattering of a facade, the final break in a chain of disappointments and hurt.

Now, as Anna stood in the bookstore, a place that symbolized her journey towards healing and independence, these memories still had the power to unsettle her. The harsh words, the silences, and the betrayal were echoes of a time when she had felt lost and diminished. She had emerged stronger, but the scars remained, sometimes aching in moments of quiet.

Anna's past relationship was a stark contrast to the life she had painstakingly built for herself and Lily. It was a reminder of her vulnerability but also of her resilience. Every time these memories resurfaced, she confronted them with a renewed understanding of her worth and strength. The bookstore, with its tranquil aisles and the scent of old books, served not just as her workplace, but as a sanctuary where she could process her past and reaffirm the life she chose to live after Ethan.

When lunchtime arrived, Anna sought refuge in the small park adjacent to the bookstore. It was a patch of green in the urban landscape, with a few benches, a fountain, and old trees that stood as silent witnesses to the ebb and flow of city life. She sat on her usual bench, a sandwich from the nearby café in one hand and her current read, "Resilience in the Shadows," in the other.

The book was more than just reading material; it was a guide and a friend. The pages spoke to her, offering wisdom and insights on how to rise above adversity. As she read, the words seemed to lift her spirit, providing a sense of understanding and a pathway to healing. The author's experiences, interwoven with practical advice, resonated with her deeply. It was as if each chapter was a steppingstone out of her own shadows, leading her towards a light that she was only beginning to see.

With each page turned, Anna felt a growing sense of empowerment. The park around her, with its gentle rustle of leaves and distant city sounds, became a backdrop to her moment of introspection and growth. It was in these quiet moments, sandwich and book in hand, that Anna found the strength to face the rest of her day, armed with newfound hope and a quiet determination to move forward, one step at a time.

As the afternoon sun began to dip lower in the sky, casting long shadows across the park, Anna closed her book and prepared to return to the bustling reality of her day. She walked back to the bookstore, her mind still echoing with the insights she had gleaned from her reading. The remainder of the afternoon passed in a blur of activity – helping customers, organizing shelves, and managing the day-to-day operations of the store.

As the clock neared closing time, Anna felt a sense of accomplishment. Despite the challenges and the emotional journey of the day, she had navigated through it with resilience and grace. She locked up the bookstore, its windows reflecting the orange hues of the setting sun, and made her way home, the familiar streets a comforting path leading her back to Lily.

The routine of the evening was a familiar dance for Anna, marked by the simple, yet essential tasks that framed her life as a single parent. The walk to Lily's school was brisk in the cool evening air, each step drawing her closer to her daughter's eager embrace. The sight of Lily running towards her with a bright, toothy grin was the highlight of Anna's day, a moment that melted away the fatigue and worries, even if just for a while.

Back at home, Anna moved through the motions of preparing dinner – chopping vegetables, simmering sauce, and boiling pasta. The kitchen was filled with the sounds and smells of cooking, a domestic symphony that was both comforting and overwhelming. Lily chattered about her day – the games she played, what she learned, and the small dramas of school life. Anna listened and engaged, her heart swelling with pride and love for her spirited daughter. Dinner was a time for them to reconnect, sharing stories about their day. Anna listened intently to Lily's school adventures, laughing at her anecdotes and offering guidance when needed. It was these everyday conversations that continued to strengthen the bond between them.

After dinner, the cleanup routine was swift, a well-practiced efficiency that had become second nature. Bath time for Lily was a splashy affair, filled with giggles and playful protests. Then came the bedtime story, a treasured ritual that had woven itself into the fabric of their lives. As Lily's eyelids grew heavy and her breathing deepened, Anna tucked her in, kissed her forehead, and whispered a goodnight full of love and silent promises.

Alone in the quiet of the living room, the weight of the day settled on Anna's shoulders. The silence of the apartment was stark, a stark contrast to the noise and bustle of the day. She slumped into the sofa, feeling the cushions embrace her tired body. The loneliness crept in like a creeping fog, cold and unwelcome. It was in these solitary moments that the void left by her past relationship felt most profound.

Reaching for her journal, a simple blue notebook that had become her confidante, Anna began to write. The pen glided across the pages, each stroke a release of thoughts and emotions that had no other outlet. She wrote about her day, about the moments of doubt and the flashes of strength. The theme of resilience, inspired by her current read, wove its way through her words. She reflected on her journey – the pain, the struggle, the endurance. Writing brought clarity and a sense of purpose, helping her to see beyond the immediate challenges.

With each word, a transformation occurred within Anna. She felt a growing sense of empowerment, a realization that she was not defined by her past or her current struggles. She was a mother doing her best, a survivor of life's harsh blows, a woman rediscovering her own strength and worth. This acknowledgment was a victory, a moment of triumph in the ongoing battle of her life.

As Anna closed her journal, a sense of peace enveloped her. She had faced another day, had navigated its challenges, and had found moments of joy and strength. Tomorrow would bring its own set of trials and triumphs, but for now, she had won a small battle against her doubts and fears.

Turning off the lamp, Anna made her way to her bedroom, the darkness a comforting blanket around her. Lying in bed, she made a silent promise to herself – to keep fighting, to keep hoping, and to never surrender to despair. The journey was long, and the path was uncertain, but she was resilient. With that thought cradling her mind, she drifted into a sleep more peaceful than she had known in a long time, ready to face whatever tomorrow would bring.

Chapter 2:

"The Echoes of the Past"

On a crisp autumn morning, the world outside just beginning to stir as Anna finds herself sitting in the waiting room of a therapist's office. It's a small, cozy space, with soft pastel walls and a bookshelf filled with volumes on psychology and self-help. The sound of a gentle fountain in the corner offers a soothing backdrop but does little to calm Anna's nerves. She's perched on the edge of a plush armchair, her hands clasped tightly in her lap. The decision to seek therapy had been a difficult one, fraught with apprehension and second-guessing, but deep down, Anna knows it's a crucial step in her journey.

As Anna enters Dr. Sarah Jennings' office, she finds herself enveloped in a space that seems designed for comfort and introspection. Dr. Jennings, standing by her desk to welcome Anna, embodies a presence that is both professional and nurturing. She is a woman in her early fifties, with a gentle face framed by soft, shoulder-length hair that shows hints of silver. Her eyes, a deep shade of hazel, reflect a depth of understanding and compassion that immediately puts Anna at ease.

Dr. Jennings is dressed in a manner that strikes a balance between professional and approachable. She wears a smart, yet not overly formal, blouse in a soothing shade of blue, paired with tailored trousers. Her attire complements the calm and inviting atmosphere of the office. A pair of simple, elegant glasses rests on the bridge of her nose, and she occasionally glances over them as she speaks, lending her an air of thoughtful attentiveness.

Around her neck, Dr. Jennings wears a delicate chain with a small pendant, which catches the light as she moves. Her overall demeanor is one of quiet confidence and warmth. As she gestures towards the seating area, her movements are graceful and considered, indicating a person who is fully present in the moment and attentive to the needs of her clients.

The therapist's office, with its soft color palette, comfortable furnishings, and shelves lined with books and therapeutic tools, reflects Dr. Jennings' approach to her work – a blend of professionalism, warmth, and dedication to providing a safe, supportive space for her clients. As Anna takes a seat, she feels a sense of safety, a feeling that in this space, under Dr. Jennings' care, she can explore her thoughts and emotions without judgment.

As they begin the session, Dr. Jennings' gentle probing steers Anna back through the years, towards memories long buried under layers of pain and resilience. Anna finds herself recounting her relationship with her ex-partner, each memory surfacing like a photograph faded with time. The scene seamlessly transitions into flashbacks.

One flashback shows a younger Anna, laughing and sharing a tender moment with her partner, a stark contrast to the later scenes of cold silences and harsh words that shattered her belief in their love. These memories are interspersed with the present, where Anna sits in the therapy room, her face reflecting the turmoil of emotions these recollections stir up.

Back in the present, within the safe confines of Dr. Sarah Jennings' office, the therapy session unfolds with a delicate and thoughtful pace. Dr. Jennings, with a practiced hand, gently steers the conversation, guiding Anna through the intricate pathways of her past experiences and their impact on her current life.

Sitting across from Anna, Dr. Jennings maintains a posture that is both attentive and non-intrusive. Her approach is methodical yet empathetic, as she encourages Anna to explore the depths of her emotions and the memories that have long cast shadows in her mind. She listens intently, her expressions one of understanding and concern, nodding encouragingly as Anna speaks.

"Let's talk about how these experiences have shaped you," Dr. Jennings suggests softly, her voice a steady anchor in the flux of emotions that Anna navigates. She leads Anna to reflect not just on the events themselves, but on the emotional responses they elicited – the pain, the resilience, and the gradual journey towards healing.

As Anna delves into her past, Dr. Jennings interjects with thoughtful questions that probe deeper into the heart of Anna's experiences. "How did you feel when that happened?" "What thoughts go through your mind when you remember these events?" These questions, though challenging, help Anna to untangle the complex tapestry of her emotions, to lay bare the fears, doubts, and strengths that have been intertwined in her story.

Throughout the session, Dr. Jennings is careful to validate Anna's feelings. She offers words of understanding and empathy, acknowledging the validity of Anna's emotions and experiences. "It's completely understandable to feel that way," she affirms, her tone validating and reassuring. Yet, she also gently nudges Anna towards a perspective of growth and understanding, encouraging her to view her experiences not just as sources of pain, but also as steppingstones to a stronger self.

"Consider how these challenges have contributed to the person you are today," Dr. Jennings advises, guiding Anna towards recognizing her own resilience and growth. She encourages Anna to acknowledge her progress, the steps she has taken to rebuild and move forward, and the inner strength she has harnessed along the way.

As the session nears its end, Anna feels a mixture of emotional exhaustion and clarity. Dr. Jennings' skillful guidance has helped her to confront and articulate feelings that were often too complex to untangle alone. She leaves the session with a sense of catharsis and a deeper understanding of her journey, equipped with insights that offer a foundation for continued healing and growth.

Anna's initial hesitance gradually gives way to a hesitant openness. She starts to articulate feelings she hadn't fully acknowledged before – the sense of loss, the erosion of trust, and the impact of the emotional scars left behind.

As the session ends, Anna feels a profound exhaustion, yet there's an undercurrent of something new - perhaps the beginnings of healing. Dr. Jennings offers some words of encouragement, reminding Anna that this is just the first step in her journey of recovery. She emphasizes that healing is not linear, and that it's okay to feel a range of emotions.

Anna leaves the therapist's office with a mix of emotions. She feels vulnerable yet empowered, having taken the first, difficult step in confronting her past. As she steps outside, the cool air hits her, and she takes a deep, steadying breath, feeling a small sense of achievement in her heart.

Post-therapy, Anna steps out into the world feeling as though she's crossed an invisible yet significant barrier. The therapy session, intense and revealing, had left her emotionally drained, yet there's an undercurrent of relief, like a storm that had passed, leaving the air clearer.

She finds herself walking almost instinctively to a nearby park, a small haven of nature amidst the city's concrete landscape. The park is a mosaic of green lawns, winding paths, and old trees whose leaves are just beginning to turn the golden hues of autumn. She selects a secluded bench under a sprawling oak tree, its leaves rustling softly in the gentle breeze, a natural symphony that's soothing and grounding.

Sitting there, Anna allows herself to fully process the therapy session. The therapist's office had been a safe space to unlock and sift through the painful memories of her past relationship. Now, in the solitude of the park, she starts to piece together how these experiences have shaped her.

She reflects on the patterns that had emerged during her conversations with Dr. Jennings – the cycle of emotional abuse she endured, the subtle erosion of her self-esteem, and how she had rationalized the unacceptable behavior of her partner. It's a painful realization, understanding how the abuse had insinuated itself into the fabric of her being, influencing her decisions and her view of the world.

In her moments of reflection, Anna begins to piece together how the deeply ingrained patterns from her past have subtly, yet significantly, woven themselves into the fabric of her day-to-day life. Her tendency to avoid confrontation, a behavior borne from years of walking on eggshells in her previous relationship, had often led her to retreat in situations where her voice needed to be heard. Whether it was in personal relationships or professional settings, this aversion to conflict had sometimes seen her rights overlooked or her needs unmet.

Anna also recognizes her habit of second-guessing her decisions, a direct result of the constant undermining she had experienced. This self-doubt had infiltrated many areas of her life, from minor choices like what to wear to major decisions like how to raise Lily or manage her career. It often left her feeling indecisive and insecure, eroding her confidence and making her question her own judgment and intuition.

Moreover, her struggle to fully trust others, a defensive mechanism developed to protect herself from further hurt, had inadvertently created barriers in forming deeper connections. This wariness had sometimes been misinterpreted as aloofness or lack of interest, holding her back from potential friendships and opportunities for support.

However, as Anna contemplates these patterns, she realizes the power in recognizing them. It's a moment of stark clarity that brings with it a sense of empowerment. Understanding these ingrained behaviors is the first crucial step towards changing them. By acknowledging these patterns, Anna can begin to consciously address them, to actively work on being more assertive, trusting her decisions, and gradually opening herself up to trusting relationships.

This recognition also brings a sense of hope and possibility. Anna understands that change is a process, one that requires time, patience, and often, guidance. But the mere act of identifying these patterns is a significant stride in her journey towards healing and growth. It gives her a roadmap for the aspects of her life she wishes to improve, turning her past experiences into lessons for a more empowered future.

As she moves forward, Anna feels a renewed sense of control over her life. She is no longer an unwitting passenger to her subconscious behaviors. Instead, she is now an active participant in reshaping her life, armed with the awareness and determination to break free from the remnants of her past that have held her back.

As she sits, lost in thought, the park around her buzzes with life. Children play on the nearby grass, their laughter a balm to her heavy heart. Couples walk hand in hand, and joggers pass by in their own rhythms. This tapestry of life happening all around her makes Anna feel both small and yet part of something larger. It's a reminder that everyone has their battles, their histories, their paths to healing.

Gradually, the sun begins its descent, casting long shadows across the park. The quality of light changes, turning softer, warmer. Anna watches this transition, feeling a kinship with the day's end. Like the day, she too has journeyed through light and darkness, and like the approaching night, she too is moving into a space of rest and reflection.

She rises from the bench, feeling a little steadier, a little more resolved. The therapy session and the subsequent reflection have been challenging, but Anna feels a sense of accomplishment. She has confronted her past, and in doing so, has taken a definitive step towards a future where she is no longer defined by it.

As Anna leaves the park, the first stars begin to appear in the evening sky, tiny beacons of light in the growing dusk. They remind her that even in darkness, there is beauty and hope. With a renewed sense of purpose, Anna heads home, ready to face whatever challenges and triumphs tomorrow might bring.

Anna, galvanized by her therapy session, decides to take a proactive role in her healing journey. She starts by turning to the vast expanse of resources available in books and online. Her apartment, once a quiet reflection of her solitary life, begins to fill with the soft rustle of pages and the gentle tapping of her keyboard as she delves into research.

One evening, Anna sits at her small dining table, now repurposed as her research station. Around her are scattered books with titles like "Healing from Trauma" and "The Power of Now." Her laptop is open to a webpage on coping mechanisms for trauma survivors. She absorbs the information, highlighting passages and taking notes. It's a new world for her, one where terms like 'mindfulness' and 'grounding exercises' start to become familiar.

One of the first techniques Anna decides to try is journaling, a practice she's already familiar with but now approaches with a renewed perspective. Instead of merely chronicling her day or outlining her emotions, she begins to use her journal as a proactive tool for healing and self-discovery. For Anna, a survivor of trauma, this shift in her journaling practice becomes incredibly beneficial. It transforms into a haven within its pages, where she can openly confront her fears and anxieties without judgment. Here, she can process her experiences in a private, controlled environment, allowing her to unpack the complex layers of her emotions at her own pace.

Journaling becomes a medium for Anna to track her progress over time, offering tangible evidence of her healing journey and personal growth. She celebrates her successes, no matter how small, which bolsters her self-esteem and reinforces her resilience. Moreover, journaling helps her to articulate her dreams and future aspirations, a step that seems particularly empowering, considering her past where such hopes were often overshadowed by her traumatic experiences.

Through this practice, Anna finds not only a method of coping but also a powerful way of reclaiming her narrative. It enables her to reflect on her feelings and experiences from a place of safety and control, which is crucial for someone healing from trauma. The act of writing helps her to externalize what she has internalized for so long, bringing clarity and understanding to her thoughts and emotions. In this way, journaling becomes a key component of Anna's journey towards recovery and self-empowerment.

Another technique that Anna discovers and incorporates into her healing journey is mindfulness, particularly through the practice of meditation. As a survivor of trauma, this approach proves to be significantly beneficial for her. She begins with just a few minutes each day, using guided meditation apps, which come highly recommended by various online support forums. Initially, Anna finds these meditation sessions challenging, as she struggles to maintain focus and quiet the persistent thoughts that often flood her mind. However, over time, these brief periods of meditation gradually transform into a profound source of peace and clarity.

For Anna, the practice of meditation becomes a vital tool in managing the aftereffects of her trauma. It teaches her to be present in the moment, a skill that is especially valuable when past traumas tend to disrupt the present. She learns the art of observing her thoughts without judgment, a practice that helps her to detach from negative patterns of thinking that were previously overwhelming. This mindful observation allows her to recognize and gently set aside intrusive memories and anxiety, giving her a sense of control over her mental space.

Moreover, meditation provides Anna with a much-needed sense of calm amidst the chaos of daily life. The tranquility she achieves during these sessions acts as a counterbalance to the stress and emotional turbulence that can arise from past traumatic experiences. This newfound calmness extends beyond her meditation practice, helping her to approach her day-to-day challenges with a more centered and peaceful mindset.

As a survivor of trauma, these moments of mindfulness and meditation become essential in Anna's journey towards healing. They offer her a sanctuary, a place of refuge where she can retreat to find balance and tranquility. The regular practice of meditation not only aids in reducing symptoms of stress and anxiety but also empowers Anna with greater emotional resilience, enhancing her overall well-being and capacity to heal from her past.

Another technique that Anna discovers and incorporates into her healing journey is mindfulness, particularly through the practice of meditation. As a survivor of trauma, this approach proves to be significantly beneficial for her. She begins with just a few minutes each day, using guided meditation apps, which come highly recommended by various online support forums. Initially, Anna finds these meditation sessions challenging, as she struggles to maintain focus and quiet the persistent thoughts that often flood her mind. However, over time, these brief periods of meditation gradually transform into a profound source of peace and clarity.

For Anna, the practice of meditation becomes a vital tool in managing the aftereffects of her trauma. It teaches her to be present in the moment, a skill that is especially valuable when past traumas tend to disrupt the present. She learns the art of observing her thoughts without judgment, a practice that helps her to detach from negative patterns of thinking that were previously overwhelming. This mindful observation allows her to recognize and gently set aside intrusive memories and anxiety, giving her a sense of control over her mental space.

Moreover, meditation provides Anna with a much-needed sense of calm amidst the chaos of daily life. The tranquility she achieves during these sessions acts as a counterbalance to the stress and emotional turbulence that can arise from past traumatic experiences. This newfound calmness extends beyond her meditation practice, helping her to approach her day-to-day challenges with a more centered and peaceful mindset.

As a survivor of trauma, these moments of mindfulness and meditation become essential in Anna's journey towards healing. They offer her a sanctuary, a place of refuge where she can retreat to find balance and tranquility. The regular practice of meditation not only aids in reducing symptoms of stress and anxiety but also empowers Anna with greater emotional resilience, enhancing her overall well-being and capacity to heal from her past.

Anna's exploration of grounding exercises marks a significant addition to her toolkit for managing the aftereffects of trauma. These practical techniques become crucial for her, especially during times of stress or when memories of past trauma unexpectedly resurface. Among these methods, she finds solace in the '5-4-3-2-1' technique, which involves identifying five things she can see, four she can touch, three she can hear, two she can smell, and one she can taste. For someone who has experienced trauma, the benefits of such grounding exercises are manifold.

Firstly, grounding techniques like the '5-4-3-2-1' exercise provide immediate relief during moments of acute stress or anxiety, which are not uncommon for survivors of trauma. By focusing on her immediate sensory experiences, Anna is able to pull her attention away from distressing thoughts or flashbacks and anchor herself firmly in the present moment. This shift in focus acts as a powerful tool to interrupt overwhelming emotions or panic, offering a way to stabilize her mental state.

Moreover, these grounding exercises enhance Anna's sense of control. Trauma can often leave individuals feeling powerless over their thoughts and emotions. Grounding techniques empower her to actively manage her response to triggers or heightened stress, reinforcing her autonomy over her mental and emotional well-being.

Practicing grounding also helps Anna to build resilience against the intrusion of traumatic memories. Over time, as she becomes more adept at these techniques, she finds that she can more effectively manage her reactions to potential triggers. This ability to self-regulate is particularly beneficial for trauma survivors, as it fosters a sense of safety and security within themselves, regardless of external circumstances.

Furthermore, grounding techniques contribute to Anna's overall healing process. By regularly practicing these exercises, she cultivates a habit of mindfulness and presence. This habit not only aids in managing symptoms associated with trauma but also contributes to a broader sense of emotional balance and well-being.

In essence, grounding exercises become a lifeline for Anna, offering a practical and immediate means to regain composure and presence. As she integrates these techniques into her daily life, they become a symbol of her ongoing journey towards recovery and a testament to her resilience in the face of life's challenges.

As Anna continues her journey, these techniques start to weave into the fabric of her daily routine. Journaling becomes her nightly ritual, a time to decompress and reflect. Mindfulness finds its way into various moments of her day, from mindful breathing during her commute to being fully present with Lily. Grounding exercises become her go-to strategy in managing moments of anxiety or flashbacks.

Through this journey of discovery and learning, Anna feels a growing sense of control over her healing process. She understands that while the road to recovery is not straightforward and is fraught with challenges, she now has tools to help her navigate it. This knowledge empowers her, providing a sense of hope and agency that she hadn't felt in a long time.

With each day, Anna becomes more adept at using these techniques. They become her companions in the journey of healing, guiding her towards a future where she is not just surviving, but thriving.
The scene unfolds on a day where the world outside mirrors Anna's internal state: gray, overcast, and imbued with an unshakeable sense of melancholy. As Anna awakens, she is immediately greeted by a pervasive feeling of unease. It's an intangible, nebulous sensation, one that doesn't point to a

specific worry or event, yet it envelops her with a sense of discomfort that is hard to ignore.

As she progresses through her morning routine, the quiet of the apartment seems to amplify her feelings. The simple act of brewing her coffee, once a cherished ritual, unexpectedly becomes a trigger. The rich aroma, which usually brings a sense of comfort and normalcy, today evokes a poignant reminder of mornings spent with her ex-partner. These memories, unbidden and intrusive, cast a shadow over the comforting routine, tainting it with a sense of loss and nostalgia.

The triggers don't stop there. As Anna turns on the radio to lighten the mood, a familiar song begins to play. It's a melody intertwined with her past, a soundtrack to moments once filled with happiness but now tinged with sorrow. The song conjures a flood of bittersweet memories, each note a reminder of what was and what has been lost. For a moment, Anna is paralyzed by the flood of emotions, standing motionless in the kitchen, caught in the grip of the past.

She attempts to break free from the grip of these memories, to push them aside and focus on the day ahead. But the feelings are stubborn, clinging to her with a persistence that is both frustrating and disheartening. It's as though the shadows of her past are determined to make their presence known, invading the peace of her present.

This morning's experience underscores the unpredictable nature of triggers for someone who has experienced trauma or loss. They can be unexpected and seemingly inconsequential things - a scent, a sound, an object - yet their impact is profound. They have the power to transport one back to a different time and place, eliciting a spectrum of emotions that can be challenging to navigate.

For Anna, this day starts as a stark reminder of the complex journey of healing and recovery. It shows that while she has made significant strides, the path is not linear, and some days will be harder than others. It's a day that tests her resilience, a day where she must once again gather her strength and use the tools she has learned - mindfulness, journaling, and grounding exercises - to bring herself back to the present and find light amidst the shadows.

The Onset of a Flashback

While at work in the bookstore, immersed in the familiar task of organizing the new arrivals section, Anna encounters a trigger that catapults her back to a darker time. A customer, browsing nearby, strikes up a casual conversation with her. They chat amiably at first, but then the customer, unaware of Anna's past, makes an offhand comment about relationships. "It's all about give and take, isn't it? Sometimes, you just must endure the bad to get to the good," they say with a light-hearted laugh.

This seemingly innocent remark hits Anna like a physical blow. In an instant, her surroundings – the rows of books, the scent of paper and ink, the gentle hum of the bookstore – fade into the background. She is transported back in time, reliving a moment from her past relationship that she has struggled to forget.

In this flashback, Anna is during a heated argument with her ex-partner, Ethan. She can almost hear his voice, sharp and accusatory, see his face contorted in anger. She remembers the feeling of walking on eggshells, trying to placate him, to make things right. The memory is so vivid that for a moment, it's as though she's there again, trapped in that cycle of tension and despair.

Back in the present, Anna's physiological response to the flashback is immediate and intense. Her heart races, pounding against her chest, a stark reminder of the fear and anxiety she once felt. Her breathing becomes shallow and rapid, as if she's struggling to catch her breath during that long-ago argument. The bookstore seems to spin around her, the edges of her vision blurring as a wave of dizziness washes over her.

For a few harrowing moments, Anna is caught in the grip of the flashback, her mind struggling to reconcile the past with the present. The sounds of the bookstore return to her ears in a disjointed cacophony, adding to her disorientation. She grips the edge of a bookshelf, grounding herself, using the solid feel of the wood under her fingers as an anchor to the here and now.

Gradually, the vividness of the flashback begins to fade. The bookstore swims back into focus, the customer's concerned face coming into view. Anna takes a deep breath, using the grounding techniques she has learned. She focuses on her immediate environment – the books in her hands, the steady rhythm of her breathing, the gentle hum of the bookstore – to pull herself back from the precipice of the past.

This incident at the bookstore is a stark reminder of the power of triggers and the impact they can have, even in seemingly safe and familiar environments. It underscores the ongoing nature of Anna's journey through healing, a path marked by moments of both vulnerability and strength.

Using Grounding Techniques

Recognizing the signs of a flashback, Anna excuses herself and finds a quiet corner in the store's small back office. She closes her eyes and focuses on her breathing, trying to steady the rapid rise and fall of her chest. She recalls the grounding exercise – the '5-4-3-2-1' technique – and begins to anchor herself in the present.

- **Five things she can see**: She opens her eyes and names five things she can see around her – a stack of books, a potted plant, a coffee cup, a calendar on the wall, and a small painting.
- **Four things she can touch**: She feels the smooth surface of the desk, the rough texture of her jeans, the cool metal of her necklace, and the soft fabric of her sweater.
- **Three things she can hear**: She listens and identifies the sound of distant traffic, the hum of the air conditioner, and the faint rustle of pages from someone browsing in the store.
- **Two things she can smell**: She concentrates and smells the lingering scent of her morning coffee and the musty aroma of old books.
- **One thing she can taste**: She takes a sip of water from her bottle, focusing on the simple act of drinking and the sensation of coolness.

As Anna goes through each step, her racing thoughts begin to slow, her breathing evens out, and the tightness in her chest loosens. The vividness of the flashback recedes, losing its grip on her. She feels more grounded, more in control.

Reflection and Resilience

flashback, her feelings, and how she managed to cope. This act of writing is cathartic, allowing her to process her emotions and recognize her resilience.

Anna understands that healing is a journey with many layers, and today she peeled back another layer. There will be more challenges ahead, but she's equipped with tools and a growing confidence in her ability to face them. As she turns off the light and goes to bed, she feels a quiet strength within her. Despite the day's struggles, she is moving forward, one step at a time.

As Anna's journey of healing and self-discovery progresses, she becomes increasingly aware of the transformative power of sharing her experiences. On a Thursday evening, a time she has come to anticipate and value deeply. She finds herself at a local support group meeting for survivors of abusive relationships, a gathering that takes place in a modest community center. The building, though nondescript from the outside, holds a special significance for those who enter its doors. Inside, it transforms into a sanctuary, a place of understanding, healing, and collective strength.

The community center's meeting room is simple yet welcoming. Chairs are arranged in a circle, fostering a sense of equality and openness among the attendees. The walls are adorned with posters and artwork, some created by members of the group, symbolizing hope and resilience. Soft lighting casts a gentle glow, creating an atmosphere that is both comforting and safe.

As Anna takes her seat, she is greeted by familiar faces. Over the weeks, these individuals have become more than just fellow attendees; they have become her allies, confidants, and friends. Each person there shares a unique yet interconnected story of struggle and survival, creating a tapestry of experiences that resonate deeply with Anna.

The support group is facilitated by a counselor who guides the discussions with a gentle hand, ensuring that each voice is heard and respected. As members share their stories, Anna listens intently, finding pieces of her own story reflected in theirs. There's a profound sense of solidarity in the room, an unspoken understanding that each person's journey, while uniquely their own, is also part of a collective narrative of overcoming and rebuilding.

When it's her turn to share, Anna speaks from the heart. She talks about her past relationship, the challenges she faced, and her journey towards healing. As she speaks, her voice is steady but laden with emotion. She articulates her fears, her moments of doubt, and her triumphs, however small they may seem. In sharing her story, Anna feels a weightlifting from her shoulders. The act of speaking her truth in a supportive, non-judgmental environment is cathartic and empowering.

The support group provides more than just a platform for sharing; it offers validation and understanding. It reassures Anna that she is not alone in her experiences. The group's empathy and shared wisdom are invaluable, offering new perspectives and coping strategies. They discuss practical ways to handle triggers, rebuild trust, and nurture self-esteem – discussions that are both enlightening and deeply affirming.

As the meeting draws to a close, Anna feels a renewed sense of hope and connection. The support group has become an integral part of her healing process, a regular reminder of her strength and the progress she has made. It's a place where her experiences are validated, her feelings are respected, and her journey towards a brighter, healthier future is actively supported.

In the shared stories and collective strength of the group, Anna finds not just comfort, but a powerful impetus to continue moving forward. She leaves the community center that evening with a sense of belonging and a renewed conviction in her path to recovery. The support group, once just a place to seek help, has now become a beacon of hope and a source of profound personal growth.

As Anna opens, the room is enveloped in a profound silence, a collective holding of breath as her story unfolds. There are nods of understanding, eyes glistening with unshed tears, and gentle gestures of support. In this moment, Anna feels a deep connection with the group, a bond forged through shared pain and resilience.

When she finishes, Laura thanks her for her bravery. Others in the group share words of encouragement, some recounting how parts of Anna's story mirror their own. This moment of sharing becomes a cathartic release for Anna, a lifting of the burden she's carried alone for so long.

Post-meeting, Anna feels emotionally raw but also strangely light. It's as if voicing her story has started to loosen the chains of her past. She realizes that her story, once a source of pain, has become a testament to her strength. By sharing it, she's not only helping herself but also offering hope to others.

On her way home, under the starlit sky, Anna reflects on the power of vulnerability and connection. She understands that her healing journey is not just about individual therapy and coping strategies, but also about community and shared healing.

Anna opening up about her past is a pivotal point in her journey. It highlights the importance of community and shared experiences in the healing process. It's a powerful testament to the strength found in vulnerability and the first step towards breaking the cycle of silence and isolation.

The night has wrapped the world outside in a blanket of silence, punctuated only by the occasional distant siren or the soft whisper of wind against the windows. Inside, the apartment is dimly lit, a single lamp casting a warm glow over the living room. Lily, Anna's beacon of light and joy, is sound asleep in her room, her gentle breathing a rhythmic lullaby in the quiet space.

Anna sits at her small dining table, now transformed into a makeshift sanctuary for reflection and writing. Her journal, a plain blue notebook that has become a repository of her deepest thoughts and feelings, lies open in front of her. A pen is poised in her hand, ready to transcribe the tumult of emotions and revelations from her heart onto the paper.

As Anna begins to write, her words flow with an honesty and clarity that surprises even her. She writes about her therapy session, the support group meeting, and the momentous act of sharing her story with strangers who quickly became companions in her journey of healing. She reflects on the pain and vulnerability she felt, and how speaking her truth had been both terrifying and liberating.

She journals about the breakthroughs and the setbacks, the days when she feels like she's moving mountains, and the days when getting out of bed feels like a herculean task. In her writing, she acknowledges the complexity of her healing process, recognizing that it's neither linear nor predictable.

As she continues to write, a thread of resilience weaves through her words. Anna realizes that with every step she takes, no matter how small, she is reclaiming pieces of herself that were lost in the shadows of her past. She writes about the strength she finds in Lily's laughter, the solace in the pages of a good book, and the newfound power in her own voice.

She contemplates the journey still ahead, the unknowns and challenges that lay before her. Yet, there's an undercurrent of hope in her reflections. She writes about the support group, the sense of community she found there, and how it's helping her to not feel alone in her struggles.

As Anna closes her journal, she feels a sense of peace. The act of writing has helped her to process and understand her experiences, to see the growth in her pain, and to recognize the resilience in her response. She looks around the quiet apartment, her haven, and feels a surge of gratitude.

She turns off the lamp, plunging the room into darkness save for the moonlight streaming through the window. As she makes her way to bed, a sense of determination settles in her heart. Yes, the path of healing is fraught with challenges, but Anna now knows that she possesses the strength to face them. She whispers a promise to herself in the darkness – to continue fighting, to keep hoping, and to never lose sight of the light, even on the darkest nights.

Chapter 3:

"Steps to Strength"

Just as the first light of dawn creeps through the curtains of Anna's bedroom. The world outside is still in slumber, offering a rare, undisturbed peace. Anna is already awake, sitting cross-legged on a small, cushioned mat in the corner of her modest living room. This has become her sacred space, her sanctuary where each day begins with purpose and mindfulness.

In these precious moments of solitude, Anna engages in a mindfulness exercise. She closes her eyes, inhaling deeply, feeling the cool morning air fill her lungs. As she exhales, she visualizes releasing the stress and worries that often plague her mind. The exercise is simple yet profound; with each breath, she feels more centered, more grounded.

Surrounding her are subtle reminders of this new journey she's embarked on – a few meditation books on the nearby shelf, a small plant basking in the morning light, and the comforting presence of her journal lying on the coffee table. These items have become integral parts of her routine, each contributing to her path of healing.

Anna's focus during her meditation is on setting intentions for the day. She reflects on what she wishes to achieve, not just in terms of tasks, but also in her emotional and mental well-being. Today, her intention is to find strength in patience, to approach challenges with a calm mind, and to be present in every moment.

As the meditation session ends, Anna gently opens her eyes, taking in the soft light that now fills the room. She feels a sense of calm readiness for the day ahead. This practice of mindfulness has slowly started to shift her perspective, allowing her to approach her day with a more balanced and positive outlook.

As Anna rolls up her yoga mat, she takes a moment to stand by the window, basking in the serene morning light that bathes her apartment. Outside, the city is beginning to stir to life; the early rays of the sun reflect off the buildings, painting the skyline in hues of gold and amber. Watching the world awaken, Anna feels a parallel stirring within herself—a waking not just to the new day but also to the myriad possibilities it holds.

This moment by the window has become a cherished ritual for her. It's a time for quiet reflection, for centering herself before the hustle of the day begins. She takes a deep breath, filling her lungs with the fresh morning air that drifts in through the open window. It's a breath of renewal and determination, a physical embodiment of her readiness to embrace the day.

With her yoga session having grounded her and set a tone of calm and mindfulness, Anna moves through her morning routine with a sense of clarity and purpose. She prepares a simple yet nutritious breakfast, each step in the process a continuation of her mindful start to the day. As she eats, she thinks about her plans, mentally preparing herself for the challenges and tasks ahead.

After breakfast, she gets ready for work, choosing her outfit with care, selecting clothes that make her feel confident and comfortable. A glance in the mirror reflects a woman who has grown stronger, more resilient, with each passing day—a woman who is learning to balance the complexities of her life with grace and determination.

As Anna leaves her apartment and steps out into the morning light, the city around her is fully awake. The streets buzz with the energy of people going about their day, a symphony of urban life that she now feels a part of. She walks to the bookstore, her steps light and purposeful, her mind clear and focused.

Mid-morning at the bookstore finds Anna in her element. Surrounded by the familiar scent of books and the quiet hum of activity, she feels a deep sense of belonging. She attends to her tasks—sorting new stock, assisting customers, arranging displays—with a diligence and passion that speak of her love for her job. Each interaction with a customer, each book that passes through her hands, adds to her sense of fulfillment.

In these hours at work, Anna finds not just a job to be done, but a space where she can be herself, where her passion for literature and her desire to connect with others through stories find a harmonious expression. As she moves among the aisles, recommending books and sharing snippets of literary wisdom, she is more than just a bookstore manager; she is a curator of stories, a guide in the world of literature.

The transition from the peace of her morning routine to the dynamic environment of the bookstore is seamless for Anna. It's a reflection of her growing ability to navigate the different aspects of her life with a grounded and hopeful heart. Each moment, from the solitude of her morning yoga to the lively interactions at the bookstore, is a thread in the rich tapestry of her day, woven together with purpose and intention.

Mid-morning at the bookstore, the warm, cozy environment is buzzing with customers. The shelves, lined with stories of every conceivable genre, stand as silent sentinels to the flurry of activity. Anna is at the heart of this, navigating the aisles with a quiet efficiency, her newfound sense of calm a stark contrast to the chaos around her.

Today presents a unique challenge. A customer, visibly agitated, approaches Anna with a complaint about a book purchase. The customer's tone is sharp, their words laced with frustration. A few months ago, this confrontation would have set Anna's heart racing, her mind clouding with anxiety. But now, armed with her new coping strategies, she faces the situation with a surprising steadiness.

Anna takes a deep, grounding breath, a technique she's learned to center herself in moments of stress. She listens attentively to the customer, offering empathetic nods. Her response is calm and measured, a testament to her practice of mindfulness. She acknowledges the customer's concern without taking the agitation personally, a skill honed through her understanding of emotional resilience.

Employing a problem-solving approach, Anna offers solutions, maintaining a polite and professional demeanor. She suggests alternatives, and even though the customer remains somewhat irritable, Anna's composed handling of the situation de-escalates the tension. The customer leaves with a resolution, if not entirely satisfied, at least acknowledged and heard.

After the customer departs, Anna takes a moment to reflect on the encounter. She feels a surge of pride for having navigated the confrontation without succumbing to stress or anxiety. It's a small victory, but significant in her journey. She realizes that the techniques she's been learning are not just theoretical concepts but practical tools that empower her in real-life situations.

Throughout the rest of her shift at the bookstore, Anna's newfound resilience shines brightly, casting a glow of positivity and calm over her work environment. The challenges of the day, which in the past might have frayed her nerves, now seem to meet a more composed and centered version of herself.

The bookstore, a hub of activity and literary exploration, presents its usual array of tasks and surprises. A busy checkout line forms as customers, eager to dive into their new finds, queue up with stacks of books. In the past, the growing line might have stirred a sense of urgency in Anna, but today, she handles each transaction with a calm efficiency, her smile unwavering. Her interactions with customers are marked by genuine warmth and attentiveness, making each person feel valued and heard.

A delivery mix-up occurs midday, with several boxes of books arriving at the wrong titles. Instead of frustration, Anna approaches the situation with a problem-solving mindset. She works systematically, sorting through the orders, coordinating with the delivery service, and ensuring the correct books are on their way. Her ability to manage the situation with grace and efficiency does not go unnoticed by her colleagues.

In fact, Anna's composed demeanor has a noticeable impact on the bookstore team. Her colleagues, who are accustomed to the sometimes-frenetic pace of retail work, find her calmness contagious. They approach their own tasks with a bit more patience and a bit less stress. The atmosphere in the bookstore becomes one of collaborative effort, where challenges are met with collective problem-solving rather than panic.

Anna's role in this positive shift is subtle yet significant. She offers help to a newer colleague struggling with the inventory system, providing guidance with a gentle patience that boosts the other's confidence. In another instance, she diffuses a customer's complaint with empathetic listening and a swift, fair resolution, turning a potential conflict into a positive experience for both the customer and the store.

As her shift draws to a close, the bookstore settles into a quieter rhythm. Anna takes a moment to straighten the displays, align the books on the shelves, and ensure everything is for the next day. There's a sense of satisfaction in these closing rituals, a feeling of fulfillment in knowing she's contributed positively to the day's success.

As she locks up the store and steps out into the evening, the events of the day replay in her mind. She realizes how far she has come, how the challenges that once would have unsettled her now serve as opportunities to demonstrate her growth and resilience. Walking home, there's a spring in her step, a reflection of the inner strength she has cultivated. Today was a good day, not because it was easy, but because she faced it with a grounded heart and a hopeful spirit.

As the day comes to an end and the bookstore's doors close, Anna feels a sense of accomplishment. She's not only contributed to the store's smooth functioning but also taken another step in reinforcing her personal growth. The challenges of the day have tested her, but they've also proven her strength and the effectiveness of the coping strategies she's embraced.

illustrating Anna's application of her new skills in a challenging environment and highlighting her personal development. It shows her journey isn't just about healing from past traumas but also about building resilience and competence in handling everyday life.

in Anna's apartment on a quiet Saturday afternoon. The living room is awash with the soft glow of sunlight filtering through the curtains. Anna and her daughter, Lily, are seated at the dining table, which is now covered with an array of art supplies – colorful papers, glue, scissors, and markers. They are working on a school project for Lily, a poster about family and community.

As they work together, there's a comfortable ease between them, a contrast to the tension that often clouded their interactions in the past. Anna is more patient, more present. She listens attentively as Lily excitedly explains her ideas for the project, her words tumbling out in the enthusiastic rush of a child's imagination.

For Anna, this moment is about more than just helping with a school assignment; it's an opportunity to connect with Lily on a deeper level. She encourages Lily to express her creativity, praising her efforts, and gently guiding rather than directing. This approach reflects a shift in Anna – she's learning to balance her role as a caregiver with being a supportive, nurturing presence in her daughter's life.

As they work, Lily asks Anna about her own childhood, her school days, and her family. Anna seizes this opportunity for an open and honest conversation. She shares memories of her own childhood, some happy, some bittersweet. Lily listens, wide-eyed, absorbing the stories. Anna keeps the conversation age-appropriate but doesn't shy away from discussing some of the challenges she's faced, framing them in a way that Lily can understand.

This exchange between Anna and Lily, unfolding in the quiet warmth of their living room, blossoms into a moment of profound connection, altering the dynamics of their relationship. As Anna shares stories from her own life - tales of her younger days, her dreams, her challenges, and even the struggles that she rarely speaks of - Lily listens with a newfound understanding and maturity. It's a revelation for Lily, seeing her mother in a new light, not just as the unwavering caregiver she has always known, but as a complex individual with a rich tapestry of experiences.

For Lily, this conversation is an eye-opener. She begins to comprehend the depth and breadth of her mother's life outside of her parental role. The stories of Anna's achievements and adventures spark admiration in Lily, while the accounts of difficulties and setbacks evoke a deep sense of empathy. This new perspective helps Lily appreciate the sacrifices and choices her mother has made, fostering a deeper respect and a stronger bond between them.

On the other hand, for Anna, sharing these aspects of her life is both liberating and healing. It's a cathartic release to voice her past dreams, recount her adventures, and even delve into the darker chapters of her life's story. The act of sharing these experiences with Lily, who listens with earnest interest and sensitivity, creates a shared space of vulnerability and trust. It's a poignant realization for Anna that her daughter is growing up, capable of understanding and sharing in the complexities of her world.

This heart-to-heart becomes a crucial turning point in their relationship. The roles of mother and daughter are enriched with a newfound mutual recognition. They begin to see and appreciate each other as individuals with their own distinct journeys, yet deeply connected by their shared experiences and love.

As the evening progresses, the conversation flows naturally, covering a spectrum of topics, from light-hearted anecdotes to more profound discussions about life. They laugh together, reflect together, and in some moments, even share a comfortable silence that speaks volumes of their strengthened relationship.

This exchange marks the beginning of a new chapter in Anna and Lily's relationship, one where open communication, mutual respect, and shared understanding lay the foundation for an even stronger bond. As they eventually say goodnight, there's a sense of gratitude and love that lingers in the air – a testament to the beautiful evolution of their relationship.

Throughout the afternoon, as they cut, paste, and decorate, there's laughter and a fair share of mess, but also moments of quiet reflection. Anna finds herself opening more, sharing thoughts and feelings she would have previously kept hidden. Lily, in her own childlike way, offers comfort and understanding.

As they finish the project, admiring their handiwork, there's a sense of accomplishment and a deeper bond forged between them. Anna feels a swell of gratitude for this time with her daughter, recognizing how her journey of healing is not only improving her life but enriching Lily's as well.

Anna tucking Lily into bed that night. As she kisses her goodnight, Lily hugs her tightly and whispers, "I love you, Mommy. You're the best." Anna's eyes fill with tears of joy. These simple words from her daughter affirm the positive changes in her life, reinforcing the importance of her journey not just for herself but for Lily too.

Anna's story is a beautiful illustration of how her personal growth is positively impacting her relationship with her daughter, showcasing the transformation in their interaction and the deepening of their emotional connection.

Facing a Setback

On a brisk Tuesday morning, Anna encounters an unexpected trigger that sends her spiraling into a moment of doubt. While sorting through old boxes in her closet, aiming to declutter her space, she stumbles upon an old photograph of her with her ex-partner, taken during a happier time. The sudden flood of memories is overwhelming, bringing back a wave of emotions she thought she had moved past.

As Anna sits on the floor of her apartment, the photograph she found while cleaning resting delicately in her hands, she is enveloped by a cascade of emotions. It's an old photograph, one that captures a moment from her past, a time that now feels like a different life. In the photo, she sees a younger version of herself, smiling, carefree, and seemingly unburdened by the hardships that would later come. The image, frozen in time, is a stark reminder of the journey she has traversed, the changes she has undergone.

The surge of sadness that washes over her is profound. It's a deep, aching longing for the simplicity and innocence of the past, for the dreams and hopes she had once held so dearly. This sadness is mingled with a sense of loss, not just for what was, but for what could have been. It's a moment of mourning for a chapter of her life that closed, a part of her identity that was irrevocably altered by her experiences.

As she gazes at the photograph, the progress she thought she had made in her healing journey seems to momentarily crumble. The walls of resilience and strength she had painstakingly built appear to weaken, leaving her feeling exposed and vulnerable. It's as if the photograph has opened a floodgate of memories and feelings, some sweet, but many painful, reminding her of the fragility of her recovery.

Anna feels shaken, the emotional impact of the photograph resonating deeply. She recognizes that healing is not a linear process; there are days when the past feels like a distant memory and others, like today, when it feels all too present. The photograph in her hands is more than just a captured moment in time; it's a symbol of her complex journey, a journey marked by moments of both weakness and strength.

In this moment of vulnerability, Anna understands that healing encompasses these periods of regression, that they are a natural part of the process of coming to terms with her past. She allows herself to feel these emotions, to acknowledge the pain and the loss, understanding that feeling them is a part of moving forward.

As she sits there, immersed in her reflections, Anna begins to gather her strength once again. She gently places the photograph away, a symbolic act of acknowledging her past but not allowing it to overshadow her present. She takes a deep breath, feeling the ground beneath her, anchoring herself back to the here and now, to the life she has been rebuilding with courage and hope.

In the midst of this emotional turmoil, Anna remembers the techniques she has been learning and practicing. She takes a few deep breaths, trying to center herself. Recalling the grounding exercises from her therapy sessions, she begins to focus on her immediate surroundings – the texture of the carpet, the sound of the city outside, the sight of Lily's artwork on the fridge.

Still feeling unsettled, Anna decides to reach out to her support group. She sends a message to the group chat, explaining her encounter with the past and her current feelings. The responses are swift and filled with empathy and encouragement. Members of the group share their own experiences with similar setbacks, offering words of comfort and reminders of her strength.

Later that evening, after Lily is asleep, Anna reflects on the day's events. She realizes that healing is not a linear process; there will be moments of unexpected challenge and reminders of the past. However, she also acknowledges the importance of self-compassion and resilience. She understands that these moments of doubt do not erase her progress.

In her journal, Anna writes about the experience, detailing her emotions, her response, and how she overcame the moment. This act of writing helps her process her feelings and put the day's events into perspective. She reminds herself of the journey she is on and how far she has come.

As Anna prepares for bed, she feels a renewed sense of determination. Today's setback was tough, but it also served as a reminder of her resilience and the support system she has built. She goes to sleep with a sense of accomplishment for having navigated through a difficult day, reaffirming her commitment to her journey of healing and growth.

depicting the realistic ups and downs of Anna's journey. It shows that while healing is not always smooth, the strategies Anna has learned and the support she has cultivated are vital in helping her manage the challenges along the way.

Strengthening Bonds in the Support Group

Several weeks have indeed transformed Anna's relationship with the support group, a transition from a hesitant participant to an integral and active member. This transformation reflects the profound journey she has undertaken, one marked by personal growth and the widening of her perspective to encompass the pains and triumphs of others.

The support group meets every week in the same cozy room at the community center, a space that has become synonymous with safety and shared understanding. The room, with its soft lighting and walls adorned with inspiring quotes and artwork, creates an atmosphere of warmth and acceptance. The circle of chairs, a physical representation of their unity and equality, invites open and honest communication.

As each session unfolds, members of the group take turns sharing their experiences. These stories range from recent struggles and setbacks to victories, however small they might seem. As Anna listens, her empathy resonates deeply within her. She can relate to their stories, having walked a similar path, and her understanding of their pain and challenges is both genuine and profound.

But Anna's role in the group has evolved. She is no longer just a listener; she has become a contributor, offering words of comfort, insights from her own journey, and sometimes, when appropriate, gentle guidance. Her comments are always thoughtful and respectful, recognizing that each person's path to healing is unique.

Her growth is most evident in the way she shares her own experiences. Where once she spoke with uncertainty and pain, she now speaks with a clarity and strength that inspires others. She talks openly about her struggles, her learning, and her gradual steps towards healing, offering her story as a testament to the possibility of recovery and growth.

Anna's presence in the group has a palpable impact. Her journey serves as an encouragement to others, a living example of resilience and hope. Her ability to empathize deeply, combined with her growing confidence in sharing her own story, makes her an invaluable member of the group.

As each meeting concludes, there's a sense of collective strength and support. The group, a tapestry of different lives and experiences, is bound by a common thread of survival and healing. For Anna, the support group has become more than a place for personal healing; it's a community where she both gives and receives support, a crucial element in her journey towards wholeness.

Walking out of the community center after each meeting, Anna feels a sense of solidarity and purpose. The support group, once a daunting prospect, has now become a source of strength and a weekly reminder of how far she has come and the journey still ahead. It's a journey she no longer walks alone but alongside others who understand and share in the path of healing.

Tonight, Anna feels a newfound confidence to take on a more active role. When a new member, visibly nervous and emotional, shares her story of struggle and escape from an abusive relationship, Anna feels a strong urge to reach out. She gently offers words of encouragement, telling the new member that she's not alone and that the path to healing, though challenging, is filled with moments of empowerment and self-discovery.

Anna shares her own progress, speaking candidly about her setbacks and victories. She talks about the mindfulness techniques she's incorporated into her daily life, how journaling has helped her process her emotions, and the strength she's found in being part of this supportive community. Her words are sincere and resonate deeply with the group, providing hope and inspiration.

As the meeting progresses, it's evident that Anna's journey is having a positive impact on others. Members of the group begin to open more, sharing their fears and triumphs. Anna listens and responds, creating a dialogue that is both healing and uplifting. Her empathy and understanding, borne from her own experiences, make her an invaluable member of the group.

There's a moment where the group engages in a group exercise designed to build trust and understanding. Anna pairs up with another member, and they share their goals for the future. It's a powerful exercise that not only strengthens the bond between members but also reinforces their individual commitments to healing and growth.

Post-meeting, as Anna walks home under the starry sky, she reflects on her growing role within the group. She realizes that by helping others, she is also reinforcing her own journey of healing. The sense of community and shared experience has become a source of strength and motivation.

She acknowledges that each person's story, including her own, is a thread in the larger tapestry of shared human experiences. This realization brings a sense of belonging and purpose that extends beyond her individual struggles.

with Anna at home, feeling a sense of fulfillment and hope. The support group has become more than a place for healing; it's a space where she contributes to the wellbeing of others, finding strength in the shared journey. As she prepares for bed, she feels connected, empowered, and part of a community that is collectively moving towards a brighter, healthier future.

with Anna in the quietude of her apartment, the only sounds being the distant hum of the city and the gentle ticking of the wall clock. It's late, and the apartment is bathed in the soft light of a single lamp. Anna is seated at her dining table, now transformed into her personal reflective space, with her journal open in front of her.

The pages of the journal are filled with Anna's neat handwriting, chronicling her journey of healing and growth. She begins to write about her recent experiences, the words flowing onto the page with an ease born from regular practice. She writes about the challenges she's faced, not just the external ones, but also the internal battles – the doubts, the fears, and the moments of weakness.

As she continues, her writing shifts to acknowledge her victories. She notes the successful handling of a confrontation at the bookstore, a testament to her newfound resilience. She writes about the deeper connection with her daughter Lily, how their relationship has flourished as she has become more present and open. She reflects on her increased participation in the support group, and how sharing her story and supporting others has brought a sense of purpose and belonging she hadn't felt before.

Anna pauses, her pen hovering over the page, as she reflects on the person she was when she began this journey and the person she is now. She realizes that her understanding of healing has deepened. It's not just about moving away from the past, but also about growing towards a future – her future, one that she shapes with every small step she takes.

She writes about the lessons she's learned – the importance of self-care, the strength in vulnerability, and the power of community. She acknowledges that the journey isn't over; there may be more challenges ahead, but she feels better equipped to face them.

As Anna closes her journal, she feels a sense of accomplishment. The act of writing has not only helped her process her thoughts and emotions but has also solidified her commitment to her journey. She understands that healing is an ongoing process, one that requires patience, courage, and self-compassion.

She stands up, stretching her arms above her head, feeling a release of tension. She walks over to the window, gazing out at the night sky. The stars are bright, a reminder of the vastness of the world and the infinite possibilities it holds.

Anna turning off the lamp and heading to bed. Her steps are light, carrying the weight of her experiences but also the strength of her resolve. As she slips under the covers, she feels a sense of peace. She has come a long way, and she is proud of her progress. Tomorrow is another day, another opportunity to continue her path of healing and growth.

In the quiet darkness of her room, Anna drifts off to sleep, her heart filled with hope and a quiet determination to keep moving forward, step by step, towards a brighter, stronger future.

Chapter 4:

"Bridging New Paths"

The first rays of sunlight streaming through Anna's bedroom window, casting a warm, golden glow that seems to infuse the room with energy and promise. Anna stirs awake, feeling an unusual lightness in her heart. Today marks a significant departure from her usual routine – she's about to dive into the uncharted waters of creative expression.

As the morning light filters through the curtains of her bedroom, Anna stands before her wardrobe, her mind set with a firm sense of resolve for the day ahead. She browses through her clothes, her fingers trailing over the fabrics, each piece holding memories and stories. Today, she's looking for something that not only offers comfort but also reflects her personality – a blend of resilience and a newly rediscovered sense of adventure.

She settles on an outfit that strikes the perfect balance: a soft, flowing blouse adorned with a subtle, bohemian print that speaks to her artistic side, paired with her favorite comfortable jeans. The blouse, with its vibrant patterns, reminds her of the times she felt most free and creative, a nod to the person she's striving to reconnect with. To complete the ensemble, she chooses a pair of simple, yet stylish, boots – practical for her day at the bookstore, yet with a touch of flair.

As Anna readies herself in front of the mirror, she takes a moment to really look at her reflection. There's a fleeting shadow of apprehension in her eyes, a natural response to the uncertainties and challenges of life. But more significantly, there's an undeniable spark of excitement, a visible sign of her growing confidence and optimism. It's the look of someone who has faced her fears, who is learning to embrace the unknown with a sense of hope.

Her morning routine is reflective and mindful, a time she uses not just to prepare for the day physically, but also to mentally and emotionally set her intentions. She applies her makeup with a light hand, enhancing her natural features, a symbolic act of highlighting her inner strength rather than masking her true self.

As Anna leaves her apartment, she takes a deep breath, feeling the cool morning air fill her lungs. She's ready to face whatever the day might bring. Walking to the bookstore, her mind drifts to the tasks ahead – the books to be shelved, the customers she'll meet, the quiet moments between tasks where she can lose herself in the pages of a new find. It's a day filled with potential, and she feels equipped to embrace it fully.

The transition from the solitude of her morning routine to the dynamic environment of the bookstore is smooth and almost meditative. With each step she takes, Anna feels more grounded, more present in the moment. She's not just going through the motions; she's actively living, actively choosing the course of her day. This sense of agency, hard-earned through her journey of healing and growth, is what fuels her as she pushes open the door to the bookstore, ready to start another day.

The local community arts center, the venue for the workshop, is a hub of artistic activity nestled in the heart of the city. Its exterior, a vibrant mosaic of murals and sculptures, is a visual symphony that immediately captivates Anna. She pauses for a moment, taking in the lively atmosphere, her ears tuning in to the melodic blend of laughter, chatter, and background music that escapes from the open doors.

As Anna steps inside, she's enveloped by the dynamic energy of the center. The lobby is bustling with people of all ages, some browsing art displays, others chatting animatedly about their projects. The air is rich with the smell of paint and coffee, creating an ambiance that's both welcoming and inspiring.

The workshop is held in a spacious, sunlit room at the back of the center. Long tables are set up with various art supplies – paints, brushes, canvases, and an array of crafting materials. The instructor, a woman with a radiant smile and eyes that spark with creativity, welcomes the participants with an infectious enthusiasm.

Anna finds a spot at one of the tables, her heart pounding with a mixture of nerves and exhilaration. She listens intently as the instructor explains the day's agenda, encouraging everyone to let go of their inhibitions and embrace their innate creativity.

As the workshop progresses, Anna dives into the activities. Whether it's a freeform painting exercise, a collaborative sculpture project, or an exploratory writing session, she engages with a newfound openness. With each brushstroke, word, and shared idea, Anna feels layers of self-doubt and restraint peeling away, revealing a vibrant inner world she had long suppressed.

One exercise has the participants painting their emotions. Anna stands before a blank canvas, her palette a rainbow of colors. She pauses, takes a deep breath, and lets her intuition guide her. The colors she chooses reflect the journey she's on – shades of blue for calm and resilience, vibrant yellows for hope and renewal, and streaks of red for passion and strength.

As Anna stands before the canvas, her initial hesitations and doubts slowly melt away, giving rise to a sense of freedom and self-expression that she seldom finds elsewhere. In her hand, the paintbrush becomes an extension of her inner self, each stroke a reflection of her journey and the emotions that course through her.

The room around her fades into a blur as she immerses herself completely in the act of painting. The only sounds are the soft bristles of the brush against the canvas and the rhythmic, soothing melody of her breathing. With each brushstroke, her movements grow more confident and fluid, as if the canvas is beckoning her to pour out her soul without restraint.

The colors she chooses speak volumes. Vibrant blues and passionate reds intertwine with soft pastels, creating a visual symphony that is as complex as it is beautiful. These colors represent the myriad facets of her life – the deep melancholy of her struggles, the fiery intensity of her pain, and the gentle hues of her healing and growth. The canvas becomes a vivid expression of her inner world, a world that has known both the depths of despair and the heights of triumph.

As the painting evolves, it transforms into more than just a piece of art; it becomes a testament to Anna's journey. The chaotic, bold strokes in some areas mirror the tumultuous periods of her life, while the smoother, more serene parts depict the moments of calm and clarity she has found. The way the colors blend and contrast with each other reflects her resilience – the ability to find balance and beauty amidst the chaos.

Lost in the act of creating, Anna experiences a profound connection between her art and her emotions. It's a form of therapy, a way for her to process and express feelings that are sometimes too complex to put into words. The act of painting becomes a cathartic release, an opportunity for Anna to confront and embrace her past, acknowledge her present, and paint her hopes for the future.

Eventually, as she steps back to view the nearly finished piece, a sense of accomplishment washes over her. The painting, in all its vibrant complexity, is a visual narrative of her life. It's a reminder of where she has been and a beacon of hope for where she is going. In this moment, with paint-stained hands and a heart full of emotions, Anna feels a deep sense of peace and fulfillment, knowing that through her art, she has found a powerful way to tell her story.

The workshop concludes with participants sharing their creations and stories. Anna, with a gentle nudge of encouragement from the instructor, shares her painting and the emotions it represents. The response is warm and affirming, with others expressing admiration and empathy.

As Anna leaves the arts center, her painting tucked safely under her arm, she feels a sense of accomplishment and joy. She's not only explored a new facet of her personality but also connected with her inner artist, something she never realized she possessed.

After her day of artistic exploration, Anna arrives back home, carrying with her not just the tangible results of her creativity, but also an invigorated spirit. Her mind races with ideas, each more colorful and exciting than the last, painting mental pictures of what she might try next. The experience at the workshop has opened a new chapter for her, one where she embraces her creative side more fully, finding joy and healing in the act of creation.

She eagerly anticipates sharing this newfound passion with Lily, envisioning future weekends where they both could dive into the world of artistic exploration together. The thought of bonding with her daughter over shared creative projects brings a warm smile to Anna's face. She imagines transforming a corner of their living room into a mini art studio, a space filled with colors, laughter, and the freedom to express themselves.

As night falls and the apartment grows quiet, Anna prepares for bed, her heart still brimming with the day's experiences. Lying in bed, she reflects on the day with a deep sense of gratitude. Stepping out of her comfort zone and into the art workshop was a leap of faith – one that paid off in ways she hadn't imagined. She realizes that each new path she explores, each boundary she pushes, is not just about discovering new hobbies or skills, but about building a richer, more fulfilling life for herself and for Lily.

"Making New Connections":

This newfound appreciation for artistic expression seamlessly connects to another aspect of her journey – the formation of new connections. The workshop had not only been a space for creative exploration but also a vibrant hub for meeting new people, each participant bringing their unique perspective and story to the table.

As Anna had looked around the workshop, she had seen it transform from a mere room into a lively, dynamic space buzzing with creativity and self-discovery. Canvases stood erect, eagerly waiting to be filled with stories and visions. Tables laden with art supplies, from brushes to paints to clay, beckoned the participants to shed their inhibitions and embrace their inner artists. The atmosphere was electric with the energy of potential, a reminder that every individual, including herself, was a vessel brimming with untold stories and hidden talents.

In that space, surrounded by people all embarking on their own journeys of self-expression, Anna had felt a profound sense of connection. It was a vivid reminder that creativity can be a powerful catalyst for building new relationships and enriching one's life with diverse experiences and perspectives. As Anna drifts off to sleep, she is not only contented with her personal achievements but also excited for the new connections that await her, both in her art and in her life.

The instructor, Marianne, with her flowing scarves and bohemian charm, moves through the room like a force of nature. Her enthusiasm for art is palpable, and her belief in art as a medium for healing and expression is inspiring. She addresses the group with a warm and engaging presence, encouraging them to let go of any preconceived notions about art and creativity. "Art is not just about skill," she says, "it's about expression, about tapping into parts of yourself that words can't reach."

Anna starts with a painting exercise. With a brush in hand, she hesitates for a moment, but then, inspired by Marianne's words, she lets her instincts take over. The colors she chooses are reflective of her emotions – deep blues and purples for the depth of her experiences, bright yellows and greens symbolizing growth and renewal. As her brush dances across the canvas, she feels a release, as if each stroke is unburdening her soul.

Next, there's a writing activity. Anna finds herself pouring thoughts and feelings onto paper, her words creating a narrative of her journey. It's raw and honest, and as she writes, she feels a sense of liberation. Her story, once a source of pain, now flows out of her as a testament to her resilience.

During a group project, Anna partners with David, a man with kind eyes and a gentle demeanor. As they collaborate on a mixed-media piece, they share snippets of their lives. David speaks of his own challenges, of lost paths, and newfound directions. Anna listens, finding echoes of her own experiences in his story.

Their conversation flows naturally, and Anna feels a connection that surprises her in its intensity. It's been a long time since she's had the opportunity to relate to someone who understands the nuances of rebuilding one's life. David's perspective is different, yet familiar, and in this shared creative space, their stories intertwine, offering comfort and understanding.

As the workshop draws to a close, Anna finds herself in a conversation with David, one of her fellow participants whose story and artistic expression had resonated deeply with her throughout the session. Their exchange is easy and natural, marked by a shared understanding of the therapeutic power of creativity. There's a sense of mutual respect and recognition as they discuss their artwork and the emotions it evoked.

In a moment of connection, they decide to exchange contact information. David hands Anna a small, neatly written card with his phone number and email address, and she reciprocates. This simple exchange symbolizes the beginning of a new friendship, one rooted in a shared passion for art and personal growth.

As Anna walks away from the workshop, her artwork tucked securely under her arm, she feels an overwhelming sense of accomplishment and anticipation. The workshop had been more than she had hoped for – not only reigniting her passion for creativity but also opening doors to new relationships and connections.

Her artwork, a vivid canvas of emotions and experiences, serves as a tangible reminder of the day's revelations and achievements. The colors and shapes on the canvas tell a story of her inner journey, capturing the essence of her feelings and thoughts. It's a personal masterpiece that symbolizes her path to self-discovery and healing.

Reflecting on the day, Anna feels a profound sense of gratitude. The workshop, with its atmosphere of support and creativity, had reminded her of the power of connection – how sharing experiences and emotions can create bonds that transcend mere acquaintance. It highlighted the beauty of shared experiences, especially in the context of healing and growth.

The prospect of a new friendship with David adds to her sense of optimism. Their conversations had sparked a sense of kinship, an understanding that each was on a unique but parallel path of self-exploration and recovery. Anna looks forward to the possibility of future artistic collaborations, discussions, and support in this new friendship.

As she makes her way home, her heart is light, filled with a renewed sense of purpose and the joy of creative expression. The experiences of the day have not only enriched her artistically but have also reinforced the importance of human connections in her life. In the journey of healing, she realizes, it's not just the internal discoveries that count, but also the external connections that we make along the way.

As Anna reflects on the day's experiences. She realizes that stepping out of her comfort zone and into the world of creative expression has opened new doors for her, both in terms of personal growth and in building meaningful relationships. As she prepares for the night, she feels a renewed sense of hope and excitement for what the future holds. This workshop, a simple step into the unknown, has become a bridge to new paths in her journey.

A Moment of Self-Realization

In the quiet of her apartment, Anna stands before a canvas, her fingers stained with a spectrum of paints – each color telling a story, each stroke a testament to her journey. The room around her fades into a blur as she becomes entirely engrossed in her art. The canvas is her world now, a world where she can express the inexpressible.

As her brush moves across the canvas, a vivid picture starts to take shape. The dark hues – deep blues and somber greys – form the backdrop, representing the challenges and hardships she has endured. These colors are stark, but essential, as they lay the foundation of her story. They speak of her pain, her struggles with the past, and the nights filled with doubt.

But amidst this darkness, there are bursts of vibrant colors. Fiery reds and oranges emerge, symbolizing her courage and determination to overcome obstacles. Lush greens and radiant yellows blossom on the canvas, illustrating her growth, renewal, and the rediscovery of hope. These brighter colors intertwine with the darker ones, creating a dynamic and balanced composition that mirrors Anna's own journey of healing.

Stepping back, Anna gazes at her painting. It's more than just a piece of art; it's a visual diary of her life. In this quiet moment of reflection, she sees not just the representation of her past, but also the embodiment of her present – resilient, hopeful, and alive with possibilities.

Anna realizes that this painting, this act of creation, symbolizes something profound. She's not just a survivor of her past, nor is she defined solely by her role as a mother. She's a complex individual, rich with dreams, talents, and potential. Her identity is a tapestry of her experiences, and she holds the power to shape its design.

With this realization, a sense of empowerment washes over her. Anna understands that her life is her own canvas, and she can choose the colors and the strokes to paint her future. She is reminded that there's more to her story than what has been; there's also what will be.

While Anna is cleaning her brushes, the painting drying in the background. She feels a renewed sense of purpose and excitement for life. Her journey of self-discovery and healing has led her to this point – standing on the brink of new beginnings and endless possibilities.

Chapter 5:

"Turning Points"

In the bookstore, where Anna is met with unexpected news. Mr. Thompson, the owner, announces his plans to temporarily relocate for personal reasons, leaving Anna in charge of the store. Along with this responsibility comes the task of organizing an upcoming literary festival, a significant event for the bookstore and the local community.

In the past, such a daunting responsibility might have overwhelmed Anna, triggering anxiety and self-doubt. However, the Anna of today receives this news with a mix of nervousness and excitement, buoyed by the growth she's experienced.

Anna approaches this new challenge with a methodical and thoughtful mindset. She starts by organizing a staff meeting, aiming to involve her team in the planning process. Her communication style reflects her growth – she is clear, open to suggestions, and assertive when sharing her vision for the event.

During the meeting at the bookstore, Anna finds herself fully engaged in the dynamics of team collaboration. The staff has gathered to discuss upcoming events, promotional strategies, and other routine bookstore matters. The room buzzes with the energy of ideas being shared and plans taking shape. Anna, as the manager, facilitates the meeting with a sense of purpose and inclusion.

As her colleagues present their ideas and concerns, Anna listens attentively. She values each contribution, ensuring that everyone feels heard and appreciated. Her approach to leadership is one of collaboration and respect, fostering an environment where creative ideas are welcomed, and constructive feedback is given thoughtfully.

However, the meeting is not without its challenges. A disagreement arises over the scheduling of an upcoming author event. One of the staff members, Mark, is particularly passionate about his proposal, but his vision clashes with the practical considerations raised by another colleague, Sarah. The discussion becomes animated, with voices raising and tensions mounting.

Anna, recognizing the signs of a potentially unproductive conflict, intervenes with a calm and steady demeanor. She acknowledges the merits in both Mark's creative ideas and Sarah's practical concerns, validating their points of view. Her ability to remain composed under pressure serves as a stabilizing force in the conversation.

To navigate this disagreement, Anna suggests a compromise that incorporates elements from both proposals, demonstrating her skill in problem-solving and conflict resolution. She proposes splitting the author event into two parts – one that aligns with Mark's creative vision and another that addresses Sarah's logistical concerns.

Her suggestion is met with nods of agreement, as the team recognizes the value in finding a middle ground. Anna's ability to mediate and steer the discussion towards a constructive resolution not only solves the immediate problem but also strengthens the team's dynamics. It reinforces a sense of unity, showing that even in disagreement, there can be collaboration and mutual respect.

By the end of the meeting, despite the challenges, there is a collective sense of accomplishment. The team leaves feeling energized and aligned, with clear action items and a shared vision for the upcoming events. Anna's leadership style, marked by her calm presence, empathetic listening, and effective problem-solving, has played a crucial role in turning potential conflicts into opportunities for growth and collaboration.

As planning for the literary festival progresses, Anna encounters various challenges – coordinating with authors, managing logistics, and handling marketing efforts. Each problem is met with a calm determination. She divides tasks among her team based on their strengths, showing trust in their abilities.

When an unexpected issue arises with the venue booking, Anna's problem-solving skills come to the fore. Instead of panicking, she quickly considers alternative locations, eventually securing a charming outdoor space that adds a unique touch to the event.

Anna's newfound confidence is evident in how she handles interactions with authors, publishers, and local businesses. She negotiates, promotes the event, and makes decisions with a newfound assertiveness.

Each successful interaction reinforces her confidence, a stark contrast to her previous self-doubt.

Anna stands in the bookstore after a long day of planning and organizing. She reflects on how far she's come – from a woman who once shied away from responsibility and leadership to one who embraces challenges with confidence and poise. The journey hasn't been easy, but she's proving to herself that she's capable of much more than she ever thought possible.

Deepening Family Bonds

Anna's home life, where she encounters a new challenge in her role as a mother. Lily, usually cheerful and energetic, has been unusually quiet and withdrawn. Concerned, Anna decides to approach the situation with the patience and understanding she's been cultivating.

Lily, who had been somewhat quiet and withdrawn, finally opens up to Anna about the problem she's facing at school. As they chop vegetables together for dinner, Lily hesitantly starts to share her struggle. She reveals that she's been having a hard time with her mathematics class. It's a subject that has always challenged her, but recently, the difficulty has increased significantly.

Lily explains that the new topics introduced in the class are complex and hard to grasp. She feels like she's falling behind her classmates, who seem to understand the material more easily. This sense of not keeping up has led to feelings of embarrassment, especially when she's unable to answer questions in class or when she receives lower grades on her assignments and tests.

The frustration is evident in Lily's voice as she talks about her attempts to understand the concepts. She mentions staying up late to go over her notes, but still finding herself confused and unsure. This ongoing struggle with math has started to impact her confidence, not just in the subject but in her academic abilities.

Anna listens attentively, offering both empathy and encouragement. She assures Lily that struggling with a subject doesn't diminish her overall intelligence or capabilities. Anna emphasizes the importance of asking for help when needed and suggests they could investigate additional resources or support, such as tutoring, to help Lily overcome her challenges in math.

This conversation in the kitchen, while centered around a specific academic issue, opens a deeper line of communication between Anna and Lily. It's an opportunity for Anna to provide guidance and support, and for Lily to learn that it's okay to face difficulties and seek help. This exchange strengthens their bond, reinforcing the trust and understanding that are integral to their relationship.

In the past, Anna might have immediately jumped into problem-solving mode, perhaps taking over the situation more than necessary. Now, she recognizes the importance of empowering Lily to address her own challenges. She listens attentively, acknowledging Lily's feelings without immediately offering solutions.

Anna shares her own experiences with overcoming difficulties, subtly weaving in lessons about perseverance and resilience. She emphasizes that it's okay to struggle and that seeking help is a sign of strength, not weakness.

After their brainstorming session in the kitchen, Lily feels more empowered to tackle her challenges in mathematics. With Anna's encouragement and support, they decide on a multifaceted approach to address the issue.

Firstly, Lily agrees to Anna's suggestion of finding a tutor. They plan to look for someone who can provide personalized assistance and explain the concepts in a way that might be more understandable to Lily. This one-on-one attention could offer her the targeted help she needs to grasp the more challenging aspects of her math class.

Additionally, Lily decides to take Anna's advice and speak with her math teacher. Encouraged by her mother's confidence in her, she resolves to ask for extra help or resources that might be available through the school. This step is significant for Lily as it involves not only seeking help but also advocating for herself, a skill that is important both academically and personally.

Anna also emphasizes the importance of regular practice and offers to help Lily create a structured study schedule. This would involve setting aside specific times each week for Lily to focus on math, ensuring that she's consistently working on the subject without feeling overwhelmed.

Throughout their discussion, Anna is careful to balance her role as a guide with empowering Lily to take charge of her own learning. She reassures Lily that encountering difficulties is a natural part of learning and that with effort and the right support, she can overcome this obstacle.

By the end of their conversation, Lily feels a renewed sense of hope and determination. She appreciates her mother's belief in her abilities and feels reassured by the concrete plan they have put in place. This approach not only addresses the immediate problem of her struggles in math but also helps Lily develop resilience and problem-solving skills that will serve her well in the future.

Anna and Lily are enjoying their dinner, the atmosphere lighter and more hopeful. Anna reflects on how her growth has positively impacted her parenting style. She's learning to strike a balance between guiding Lily and allowing her the space to grow and learn from her own experiences.

This moment between Anna and Lily is significant as it highlights the positive changes in their relationship. Anna's journey of self-improvement and healing is not only transforming her own life but also enabling her to be a better, more empathetic parent to Lily.

Rekindling Old Passions

As Anna continues to navigate the complexities of her life with newfound resilience, she realizes that in the midst of her struggles and responsibilities, she had set aside a part of herself – her love for music, particularly playing the guitar. This realization comes one evening as she cleans the attic and finds her old, dusty guitar in a corner. It's a poignant moment, filled with nostalgia and a sense of loss for the time gone by.

Encouraged by her recent experiences of stepping out of her comfort zone, Anna decides to rekindle her passion for music. She begins by cleaning and tuning the guitar, a process that feels symbolic, almost like she's tuning her life to a new rhythm.

Anna's love for music stems from its profound and multifaceted impact on her life. For her, music has always been more than just a collection of melodies and lyrics; it has been a companion, a source of inspiration, and a means of expression.

1. Emotional Connection: Anna has always felt a deep emotional connection to music. It has the power to evoke and amplify a wide range of emotions, from joy and hope to melancholy and introspection. Certain songs or pieces resonate with her own experiences, allowing her to feel a sense of kinship and understanding.

2. Creative Outlet: Music provides Anna with a creative outlet, a way to express feelings that might be difficult to articulate in words. Playing the guitar or immersing herself in a song allows her to channel her emotions into something tangible and beautiful, offering a sense of release and fulfillment.

3. Sense of Identity: Music has been a significant part of Anna's identity. It's something that has set her apart and given her a unique voice. Whether she's playing the guitar, writing a song, or simply losing herself in her favorite album, music is a way for her to connect with who she is and what she feels.

4. Source of Comfort and Healing: Throughout her life, especially during challenging times, music has been a source of comfort and healing for Anna. It has been a means to soothe her soul and bring her peace, acting as a therapeutic escape from the stresses and pains of life.

5. Connection to Others: Music also serves as a way for Anna to connect with others. It's a universal language that transcends barriers and brings people together. Sharing music, whether it's playing for friends or enjoying a concert, creates shared experiences and deepens her relationships.

By rekindling her passion for music and tuning her guitar, Anna is not just engaging in a hobby; she is reigniting a part of her soul that resonates with joy, creativity, and expression. It symbolizes a turning point in her life, a decision to embrace joy and passion amidst the ongoing journey of healing and self-discovery.

In the evenings, after Lily goes to bed, Anna dedicates time to her guitar. At first, her fingers fumble over the strings, the chords and melodies not as smooth as they once were. But she persists, driven by the joy and sense of peace she feels with every note.

As the days pass, her skills start to return. The music fills her apartment, a soundtrack to her journey of healing and growth. Sometimes, Lily joins her, and they sing together, turning these sessions into special bonding moments. Music becomes a conduit for expressing emotions, a language that speaks of Anna's journey, her hopes, and her dreams.

Encouraged by her progress and the joy it brings, Anna decides to share her music with others. She learns about an open mic night at a local café and, mustering her courage, signs up to perform. The night of the performance, Anna feels a mix of excitement and nerves. But once she's on stage, guitar in hand, under the soft lights of the café, she finds herself immersed in the music.

Her performance is heartfelt and receives warm applause. There's a sense of accomplishment in sharing a piece of herself with an audience, a feeling that's both exhilarating and liberating. Post-performance, several attendees compliment her, and she even receives an offer from the café owner to play there regularly.

Anna reflects on what reclaiming her love for music has brought to her life. It's not just about the joy of playing or the applause; it's about reconnecting with a part of herself that she thought she had lost. It's a testament to her growth and her ability to find happiness and fulfillment in her passions.

As Anna sits quietly, guitar in hand, contemplating the new opportunities that her rekindled passion for music might bring. This rediscovery has not only brought joy and fulfillment but also opened doors to new experiences and connections, adding another layer of richness to her life.

A Setback and Recovery

on a seemingly ordinary afternoon. Anna, while feeling a sense of accomplishment in her recent endeavors, encounters an unexpected trigger. As she sorts through some old papers, she finds a letter from her past – a reminder of her previous relationship. In the letter that Anna finds, hidden among old papers, are the echoes of a past that she has worked hard to move beyond. The letter is from her ex-partner, written during a time when their relationship seemed full of potential and hope. The words on the page, now bittersweet, are a poignant reminder of a period in her life marked by both love and subsequent heartache.

Promises: The letter contains promises that were never fulfilled, which at the time had painted a picture of a future together that was never realized. These may have included commitments of lasting companionship, mutual support, and building a life together. The promises might have been about overcoming challenges as a team, being each other's steadfast partner, or perhaps taking steps towards common goals and dreams.

Dreams: The dreams articulated in the letter likely centered around shared aspirations and plans. This could have involved specific ideas like buying a home together, traveling to places they both wanted to explore, or maybe starting a family. There might have been mentions of shared professional or personal goals, like supporting each other through career changes or joint ventures, or dreams of shared experiences and adventures that were to solidify their bond.

Finding this letter unearths a mix of emotions for Anna. On one hand, it's a stark reminder of a period in her life filled with hope and love. On the other, it brings back the pain of realizing those promises were left unkept and those dreams unfulfilled. The letter symbolizes not just a lost relationship, but a divergence from a path she once thought her life would take.

This encounter with the past, while painful, also serves as a testament to the journey Anna has undertaken since. It highlights the contrast between who she was then and who she is now – a woman who has grown stronger and more resilient in the face of life's complexities. While the letter opens old wounds, it also reaffirms Anna's progress in healing and moving forward.

The impact is immediate and intense. Anna feels a wave of emotions washing over her – sadness, regret, and a sense of loss for what could have been. Her hands tremble as she holds the letter, and for a moment, she feels as if she's taken several steps back in her journey of healing.

Recognizing the onset of these overwhelming emotions, Anna pauses. She reminds herself of the coping strategies she's learned. Taking deep, steady breaths, she practices mindfulness, focusing on her surroundings to anchor herself in the present. She acknowledges her emotions but doesn't let them consume her, a skill she's been cultivating in therapy.

Needing to process these feelings, Anna reaches out to her support group. She sends a message, sharing her experience and seeking the comfort of those who understand. The responses are swift and empathetic, offering both comfort and perspective. One member reminds her, "It's okay to visit the past, just don't stay there."

Later that evening, Anna takes time for self-reflection. She journals about the experience, pouring out her thoughts and feelings. This act of writing helps her process the emotions stirred by the letter. She writes about her pain, but also about her growth since then. She acknowledges that while her past is a part of her story, it does not define her future.

In a symbolic gesture of letting go, Anna decides to discard the letter. She tears it up, releasing the hold those memories had on her. It's a small but significant act, reinforcing her commitment to moving forward.

Anna feels a renewed sense of strength and clarity. This setback, while painful, has shown her how much she's grown. She's able to face reminders of her past without unraveling, using the tools and support systems she's put in place.

Strengthening Community Ties

As Anna continues to navigate her path of self-discovery and healing, she recognizes a growing desire to extend her journey beyond personal growth, reaching out to be an active part of her community. This newfound aspiration leads her to participate in a local community project.

The "Green Spaces" project that Anna discovers is a community-driven initiative, a movement aimed at transforming local parks and public areas into vibrant, welcoming spaces. It's an effort that resonates deeply with Anna, aligning with her growing desire to engage more actively with her community and contribute to meaningful causes.

Project Details:

- **Beautification and Revitalization:** The primary goal of "Green Spaces" is to revitalize local parks and public areas. This involves planting trees and flowers, installing benches and art installations, and cleaning up existing spaces to make them more inviting and accessible to the community.
- **Community Engagement:** A significant aspect of the project is bringing together residents from all walks of life. It's about building a sense of community and shared responsibility, encouraging people to take pride in their neighborhood. The project organizes regular weekend meetups, workshops on gardening and environmental care, and community events in the parks.
- **Sustainability Focus:** "Green Spaces" also has a strong focus on sustainability. Part of its mission is to educate the community on eco-friendly practices, promote biodiversity, and create green spaces that not only look beautiful but also contribute positively to the local ecosystem.
- **Artistic Expression:** The project invites local artists to contribute, turning parks

into canvases for artistic expression. This includes mural painting, sculpture installations, and other forms of public art that celebrate the community's culture and diversity.

Anna's Involvement: Intrigued by the project's multifaceted approach, Anna signs up to volunteer. She sees this as an opportunity to not only give back to her community but also to connect with like-minded individuals. Her enthusiasm for "Green Spaces" is fueled by her belief in the transformative power of communal effort and her passion for nature and the arts.

- **Volunteering Roles:** Anna takes on various roles within the project. She participates in the weekend gardening activities, helps with the organization of community events, and even lends a hand in some of the artistic endeavors.
- **Building Connections:** Through her involvement, Anna meets a diverse group of people – from passionate environmentalists to local artists. These interactions enrich her experience, providing her with new perspectives and

deepening her connection to her community.

- **Personal Growth:** Volunteering with "Green Spaces" also becomes a journey of personal growth for Anna. It allows her to step out of her comfort zone, learn new skills, and see the direct impact of her efforts in beautifying and nurturing the communal spaces around her.

As Anna immerses herself in the "Green Spaces" project, she finds a sense of fulfillment and joy. Her weekends spent volunteering become highlights of her weeks, offering a balance to her work life and an avenue to pursue her passions. The initiative becomes more than just a project; it's a reflection of Anna's values and a testament to her commitment to making a difference in her corner of the world.

On the day of the project, Anna arrives at the designated park, a little nervous but mostly excited. She's greeted by a diverse group of volunteers, all buzzing with energy and a shared purpose. The project leader, a spirited man named Carlos, welcomes her warmly, explaining the day's tasks which include planting flowers, painting benches, and cleaning up the pathways.

Anna throws herself into the work, feeling a sense of camaraderie with her fellow volunteers. As they dig, plant, and paint, conversations flow naturally. Anna finds herself opening about her love for nature and her recent journey towards personal growth. In turn, she hears stories from others, each unique yet bound by common threads of hope, struggle, and community spirit.

During a break, Anna finds herself chatting with a group of volunteers. They discuss the project, but also touch on deeper topics like the importance of community support and personal challenges. Anna shares insights from her own experiences, offering words of encouragement and understanding. Her openness and empathy resonate with the group, forging new connections built on mutual respect and shared experiences.

As the day progresses, the park transforms under their collective effort. What was once an overlooked space becoming a vibrant and inviting area for the community. Standing back and looking at their handiwork, Anna feels a surge of accomplishment and belonging. She realizes that this project is not just about improving a physical space; it's about building a community, fostering connections, and creating an environment where people can come together.

Anna returns home, tired but fulfilled. She reflects on the day, feeling proud of her contribution and the new relationships she's begun to form. This experience has not only allowed her to give back but has also deepened her sense of belonging and purpose within her community.

Scene 6: Reflections of Growth

Scene 11: Quiet Reflection at Home

The chapter draws to a close on a quiet evening in Anna's apartment. The events of the day have subsided into a peaceful stillness. Anna sits in her favorite armchair by the window, a cup of herbal tea in hand, gazing out at the starlit sky. The gentle hum of the city at night provides a soothing backdrop as she reflects on the journey she has undertaken.

In this tranquil setting, Anna allows herself to truly absorb the magnitude of the changes she has experienced. She thinks back to the person she was before – uncertain, overwhelmed by her past, and unsure of her place in the world. She then considers who she is now – more confident, grounded, and actively engaged in shaping her life and her community.

Scene 12: Acknowledging Her Journey

Anna's mind wanders through the various milestones of her journey. From the painful first steps of acknowledging and confronting her past, to finding her voice in the support group, to rediscovering her love for music, and now, contributing to a community project. Each experience, with its own set of challenges and triumphs, has contributed to her growth.

She reflects on the setbacks she has faced along the way – moments of doubt and reminders of her past. Yet, she recognizes that these are not signs of failure but integral parts of the healing process. They have taught her resilience, the importance of self-compassion, and the value of her support network.

Scene 13: Envisioning the Future

Looking forward, Anna feels a sense of optimism about her future. She acknowledges that the journey of self-improvement and healing is ongoing, with no definitive endpoint. However, she now views this not as a daunting prospect but as an opportunity for continuous growth and discovery.

Anna contemplates her goals and aspirations. She envisions herself not only continuing to nurture her personal passions and relationships but also playing a more active role in her community. She sees potential paths unfolding before her – perhaps furthering her involvement in community projects, exploring new creative avenues, or even using her experiences to help others on their own journeys of healing.

Closing the Chapter

The chapter concludes with Anna feeling a profound gratitude for the journey she has embarked upon. She recognizes that while the road has been and will continue to be challenging, it is also rich with opportunities for learning and growth. She feels equipped with the tools, the support, and the inner strength to face whatever lies ahead.

As Anna sets her tea cup down and prepares for bed, she feels a sense of contentment and hope. Her journey has transformed her in ways she never imagined, and she is ready to embrace whatever the future holds. The night whispers promises of new beginnings, and Anna, with a heart full of newfound purpose and resolve, steps into her dreams.

Chapter 6:

"New Horizons"

In the early hours of the morning, as the first light of dawn casts a soft glow through her kitchen window, Anna stands up from the breakfast table. She holds an empty mug that once brimmed with her morning coffee, the last few sips of which provided a quiet moment of reflection. As she places the mug in the sink, the gentle clink of ceramic against stainless steel resonates in the stillness of her apartment.

Taking a deep breath, Anna feels a profound connection with the changing season outside her window. The world is transitioning, and so is she. With each passing day, she finds herself more in tune with the rhythm of life, more aligned with her own inner changes. It's a feeling of renewal, mirroring the natural cycle of growth and transformation that surrounds her.

Moving to her small writing desk by the window, Anna opens her journal. This journal, a constant companion in her journey, has witnessed her fears, hopes, dreams, and reflections. Today, it's about looking forward. She takes her pen and begins to outline her goals and plans, each word a deliberate step toward the future she is ready to embrace. These goals span various aspects of her life – personal development, her career at the bookstore, her role as a mother, and her contributions to community projects like "Green Spaces."

As she writes, her plans begin to take shape. For her personal growth, she notes continuing her involvement in the support group and exploring more creative outlets, like the art workshop she recently attended. Professionally, she wants to implement new ideas at the bookstore, perhaps organizing more community events or expanding the store's offerings.

Anna also dedicates a part of her plan to being the best mother she can be for Lily, ensuring that she supports her daughter's academic and personal growth. This includes spending quality time together, being present and engaged in Lily's life, and fostering an environment of open communication and mutual respect.

Finally, she notes her ongoing commitment to "Green Spaces," envisioning her active participation in upcoming projects and events that will further enhance the community's green areas.

With her goals outlined, Anna feels a sense of clarity and determination. She closes her journal, ready to start her day, emboldened by the knowledge that she is actively shaping her life's path.

Anna prepares for work, her mind abuzz with the plans she's just penned down. She dresses in a manner that reflects her newfound confidence and purpose, choosing an outfit that is both professional and expressive of her personality. As she locks her apartment door and steps out, she feels a sense of anticipation for the day ahead.

On her way to the bookstore, Anna walks with a brisk, purposeful stride. She thinks about the tasks awaiting her, the customers she'll meet, and the new initiatives she plans to propose. Stepping into the bookstore, she's greeted by the familiar scent of books and the quiet hum of early morning activity. Here, in this space of stories and knowledge, Anna finds another aspect of her life where she can make a meaningful impact.

The transition from the introspection of her morning routine to the vibrant energy of the bookstore is seamless. With each step, Anna feels more connected to her goals and more grounded in her role as a bookstore manager. She's not just going through the motions; she's actively building the future she envisions, one day at a time.

Mr. Thompson, back from his absence, surveys the store with a pleased expression. The atmosphere is vibrant, the displays are more appealing, and there's a noticeable increase in customer engagement – all fruits of Anna's hard work and dedication.

Mr. Thompson calls Anna into his office, a room lined with books and mementos from his years in the business. The air is filled with a mix of anticipation and nervous excitement as Anna steps in. Mr. Thompson commends her for the exceptional job she's done, acknowledging her natural flair for management and her creative initiatives that have positively impacted the store.

He then presents Anna with a significant opportunity – a promotion to a managerial position, or perhaps the chance to lead a new project that aligns with her passions, like organizing regular community events or literary workshops at the bookstore. This recognition of her talents and efforts is a pivotal moment for Anna, symbolizing her growth not just personally, but professionally as well.

The prospect of this new role excites Anna, filling her with a sense of pride and accomplishment. However, it also brings a new set of challenges. Taking on greater responsibilities at work means she will need to find a balance with her personal life, her commitments to Lily, her involvement in community projects, and her own self-care routines.

Anna takes some time to reflect on this. She considers her options, thinking about how she can manage her time and responsibilities effectively. Drawing on her newfound resilience and the organizational skills she has honed, Anna starts to formulate a plan. She thinks about setting clear boundaries, prioritizing tasks, and perhaps even seeking additional support, like delegating certain responsibilities both at work and home.

Anna feels a surge of confidence. She's aware of the challenges ahead but feels equipped to face them. Her journey has taught her about her own strength and capabilities, and she's ready to take on this new role.

Anna steps out of Mr. Thompson's office, her mind already buzzing with ideas and plans for her new position. She feels grateful for this opportunity to grow and make a more significant impact in a place that she loves. The chapter ends with Anna sharing the news with Lily, who beams with pride and excitement for her mother. This new chapter at the bookstore is not just a professional advancement for Anna, but a testament to her journey of transformation and empowerment.

Deepening Relationship

With Anna's increased responsibilities at work, she becomes even more conscious of the time she spends with Lily. To ensure they maintain their close bond, Anna and Lily embark on a shared project – starting a small garden in their apartment balcony.

The project that Anna and Lily embark upon is the creation of a small home garden, a venture that combines their shared love for nature with a desire to beautify their living space. This initiative is not just about planting and gardening; it's a meaningful endeavor that represents growth, nurturing, and bonding.

Set on a sunny afternoon, their first step involves a visit to a local nursery, a place brimming with the potential of new life and growth. The nursery is a colorful mosaic of plants, flowers, and gardening supplies, offering a plethora of choices for their new project.

Lily's excitement is palpable as they walk through the rows of plants. Her eyes are drawn to the vibrant colors and varied textures of the flowers and herbs. She enthusiastically picks out an array of colorful blooms and fragrant herbs, each selection made with a child's innate attraction to beauty and wonder. Her choices include bright marigolds, delicate petunias, and aromatic basil and mint, adding both aesthetic appeal and practical use to their garden.

Anna, while equally enthused, takes on a more practical approach to complement Lily's creative selections. She focuses on the essentials needed to turn their vision into reality. This includes choosing the right pots that will not only hold the plants but also fit aesthetically in the spaces they have at home. She selects nutrient-rich soil, ensuring that their chosen plants have the best foundation to thrive. Anna also considers other gardening tools and supplies they might need, like watering cans, trowels, and gloves.

Together, their collaboration is a harmonious blend of Lily's creative ideas and Anna's organizational skills. Lily brings the imagination and enthusiasm, envisioning what their garden could look like, while Anna provides the structure and planning, turning those visions into actionable steps.

This project symbolizes a shared journey for Anna and Lily. It's an opportunity for them to spend quality time together, learn from each other, and create something beautiful and nurturing. The act of caring for their garden will teach Lily about responsibility and the joys of tending to living things, while for Anna, it's a chance to bond with her daughter and find joy in the simple pleasures of life.

Their day at the nursery marks the beginning of this delightful project, setting the stage for many fulfilling days of gardening and growth ahead.

As they work together on the balcony, planting and arranging, there's laughter and learning. Anna teaches Lily about caring for plants, but also takes this opportunity to draw parallels with life lessons – nurturing, patience, and the joy of watching something grow. These moments become precious to both, a time to connect not just through conversation but through shared activity.

Parallel to the deepening bond with her daughter, Anna finds herself at the cusp of a new chapter in her personal life. During one of the literary events at the bookstore, she meets Michael, a guest speaker who is an author and a professor. There's an immediate and undeniable connection – they share a love for literature, and their conversation flows effortlessly.

Michael, the guest speaker at the literary event at Anna's bookstore, is a figure who exudes both intellect and charisma. As an author and a professor, his life revolves around the world of words and ideas, passions that Anna finds deeply relatable and attractive. Michael is in his late thirties, with a career that balances academia and creative writing. He teaches literature at a local university, where he is well-regarded both by his colleagues and students for his insightful lectures and approachable nature. His published work, which includes a mix of literary fiction and essays on contemporary themes, has garnered acclaim for its depth and eloquence. His love for literature is not just a profession but a way of life, something that becomes immediately apparent in his articulate and thoughtful manner of speaking. Michael carries an air of understated confidence. He has a tall, lean build and carries himself with an ease that is both inviting and intriguing. His features are sharp, softened by a warm smile that often plays on his lips, especially when engaged in lively discussions about his favorite subjects. He has expressive eyes that light up when he talks about literature, reflecting a mind that is always exploring and analyzing.

His attire during the literary event is a balance of casual and professional – a smart blazer over a simple shirt, paired with well-fitted jeans. It's an ensemble that speaks of someone who values comfort but also takes pride in his appearance.

During their conversation at the event, Anna and Michael discover a shared love not only for literature but also for many other facets of art and culture. They find common ground in their favorite authors and genres, and their discussion naturally veers into deeper topics like the role of storytelling in society and the evolving landscape of modern literature.

The connection between them is palpable. It's not just about shared interests; it's a meeting of minds, a mutual recognition of similar values and outlooks on life. Michael listens to Anna with genuine interest, valuing her insights and experiences. For Anna, it's refreshing to find someone who not only shares her passions but also respects and engages with her perspectives.

Their interaction at the event lays the foundation for a burgeoning relationship, one that holds the promise of intellectual companionship and perhaps, in time, something deeper. As the event concludes, they both express a desire to continue their conversation, setting the stage for future meetings. For Anna, meeting Michael is a serendipitous moment, marking the beginning of a new and exciting chapter in her personal life.

In the days that follow, Anna finds herself thinking about Michael. He reaches out to her, asking if she would like to join him for coffee. Anna, who hasn't considered a romantic relationship for a long time, feels a mix of excitement and apprehension. She decides to take the chance, agreeing to meet him.

Anna and Michael's coffee date unfolds in a charming, quaint café, the kind of place where the aroma of freshly brewed coffee blends with the warmth of cozy surroundings. The café, with its rustic decor and soft background music, provides an ideal setting for a relaxed and intimate get-together. Small tables are scattered around, each offering a private nook for conversations, while gentle lighting casts a soothing ambiance.

A   s they sit across from each other, their conversation flows effortlessly. They chat about a variety of topics – from lighthearted anecdotes about their day-to-day lives to more profound discussions about their interests and aspirations. Michael shares stories that make Anna laugh, his sense of humor a delightful surprise. Anna finds herself opening up about her hobbies, her work at the bookstore, and even touches upon her love for art and gardening.

Throughout the date, Anna feels an unexpected sense of ease and connection with Michael. His demeanor is respectful and engaging, creating a space where she feels comfortable to be herself. They discover shared interests and viewpoints, and even when their opinions differ, it adds depth to their conversation, making it even more engaging.

However, amidst this pleasant experience, Anna remains cautiously aware of her own feelings and boundaries. Her past experiences have taught her the importance of moving at a pace that feels right for her. She enjoys the laughter and the shared stories, but a part of her remains mindful of the journey she's been on, the challenges she's overcome, and the independence she's worked hard to build. This mindfulness doesn't diminish her enjoyment of the date; rather, it gives her a sense of empowerment and control over her choices.

As they sip their coffee and the hours pass by, Anna appreciates the simplicity and honesty of the moment. There's no pressure or expectations, just two individuals enjoying each other's company. As they eventually say goodbye, with promises to meet again, Anna feels a flutter of happiness, coupled with the assurance that taking things slowly is the right approach for her at this stage in her life.

This coffee date with Michael marks not just a potential beginning of a new relationship but also a testament to Anna's growth. She's learning to balance her desire for connection with her need for self-care and independence. It's a delicate dance, but one that she's now more equipped and confident to navigate.

Anna reflects on these new developments in her personal life. Working on the garden project with Lily has not only strengthened their bond but also given her a sense of joy in shared accomplishments. The prospect of a new romantic relationship, while still in its nascent stages, opens up a realm of possibilities that Anna had not allowed herself to consider for a long time.

Overcoming Personal Barriers

As Anna navigates the new dynamics of her life, she encounters internal conflicts that challenge her growth. With her promotion at the bookstore, while she is outwardly confident and capable, inwardly she battles lingering doubts about her abilities to handle the increased responsibilities. She sometimes finds herself questioning if she's truly qualified for the role, a remnant of the insecurity she has worked hard to overcome.

Meanwhile, in her personal life, as her relationship with Michael begins to develop, Anna confronts fears and insecurities about opening her heart again. Memories of her past relationship occasionally surface, casting shadows of doubt over this new possibility of happiness.

Aware of these internal conflicts, Anna turns to the coping strategies she has learned. She practices mindfulness to stay grounded in the present moment, especially when doubts about her professional abilities creep in. She sets aside time each day to meditate, focusing on her breath and the sensations in her body, which helps her center her thoughts and alleviate anxiety.

Anna's journal becomes a canvas for her to express and examine her personal fears, particularly those surrounding her developing relationship with Michael. These fears are deeply rooted in her past experiences and her journey of healing and growth.

1. Fear of Repeating Past Mistakes: Having emerged from an abusive relationship, Anna harbors a fear of inadvertently finding herself in a similar situation. She worries about missing red flags or getting too involved too quickly without fully understanding a person's character.

2. Fear of Losing Independence: Anna has worked hard to rebuild her life and establish a sense of independence and self-sufficiency. The prospect of a new relationship brings with it the fear of losing this newfound autonomy. She worries about the possibility of becoming too dependent on someone else for her happiness and well-being.

3. Fear of Vulnerability: Opening up to someone new and allowing herself to be vulnerable again is a daunting prospect for Anna. Her past experiences have left her cautious about exposing her emotions and fears, concerned that this vulnerability could be taken advantage of.

4. Fear of Trusting Someone New: Trust is a significant concern for Anna. Her previous relationship's betrayal has made her wary of placing trust in someone new. She fears the risk of being hurt again if that trust is broken.

5. Fear of Impact on Her Daughter: As a mother, Anna is acutely aware of how her personal life can impact her daughter, Lily. She fears that bringing someone new into their lives might affect Lily, especially if the relationship does not work out. Anna is protective of the stable and secure environment she has created for her daughter.

In her journal, Anna confronts these fears with honesty and introspection. She acknowledges them not as weaknesses, but as natural concerns stemming from her experiences. Alongside her fears, she also writes about her hopes – for a relationship built on mutual respect and understanding, for the joy of companionship, and for the opportunity to share her life with someone who values her as she is.

Journaling allows Anna to process her emotions at her own pace, helping her balance her fears with a cautious optimism. She reflects on the lessons learned from her past, using them as a guide to navigate her future. This practice of writing becomes a therapeutic process, aiding her in her continuous journey of self-discovery and personal growth.

In addition to relying on her own strategies, Anna seeks support from her network. She has a heartfelt conversation with Mr. Thompson, expressing her fears about her new role. His reassurance and confidence in her abilities bolster her self-esteem.

Anna also turns to her support group, sharing her apprehensions about her new romantic relationship. The members, many of whom have faced similar challenges, offer empathy and advice. They remind her of her strength and how far she has come, encouraging her to embrace happiness without letting fear hold her back.

Anna is feeling a renewed sense of empowerment. Though acknowledging her fears and insecurities is challenging, confronting them head-on reaffirms her commitment to personal growth. She realizes that these inner conflicts are part of her journey and that facing them is crucial to moving forward.

Anna ends the day with a quiet moment of reflection, acknowledging that while the path to growth is never without obstacles, she possesses the strength, tools, and support to overcome them. She goes to bed with a sense of peace, knowing that each step she takes, even the small ones, is a stride towards a stronger, more confident self.

Giving Back

Inspired by her journey of self-discovery and healing, and buoyed by her recent successes, Anna feels a strong desire to give back to the community that has supported her through her challenges. She recognizes that her experiences, both struggles and triumphs, could be invaluable to others facing similar situations.

After much contemplation, Anna decides to initiate a project that aligns with her experiences and passions. She plans to start a series of workshops titled "Creative Healing," designed to help individuals who have gone through personal traumas and challenges, using creative expression as a tool for healing and personal growth.

Anna's project, which she titles "Creative Healing," is a heartfelt initiative that combines her own journey of healing with her passion for creative expression. This series of workshops is designed to offer support and a creative outlet to individuals who have experienced personal traumas and challenges. Anna envisions "Creative Healing" as a space where art, in its various forms, becomes a medium for processing emotions, fostering resilience, and promoting personal growth.

Key Aspects of the 'Creative Healing' Workshops:

1. **Artistic Expression:** The workshops provide a variety of artistic mediums – such as painting, writing, music, and crafts – for participants to explore. These activities are not about creating perfect art but about using creativity as a tool for self-expression and reflection.

2. **Safe and Supportive Environment:** Recognizing the vulnerability that comes with sharing personal experiences, Anna ensures that the workshops are conducted in a safe, welcoming, and non-judgmental environment. This space allows participants to feel comfortable expressing themselves and sharing their stories if they choose to.

3. **Guided Sessions:** Each workshop is structured yet flexible, with guidance provided by Anna or guest facilitators who are professionals in therapeutic art practices. These facilitators help guide the creative activities, ensuring they are tailored to the needs of the participants.

4. **Focus on Healing and Growth:** The core aim of these workshops is to aid in the healing process. They are based on the premise that

engaging in creative activities can provide emotional relief, help process trauma, and foster a sense of peace and well-being.

5. **Community Building:** "Creative Healing" also aims to build a community of support among participants. By bringing together people who have faced similar challenges, the workshops create opportunities for connection, empathy, and mutual support.

6. **Resource and Skill Development:** Apart from creative activities, the workshops also include sessions on developing coping strategies, resilience skills, and self-care practices. This holistic approach ensures that participants can continue their journey of healing and growth beyond the workshops.

Anna's decision to start this project is deeply personal. It stems from her own experiences with trauma and the solace she found in creative expression. She understands firsthand the therapeutic power of creativity and wants to extend that opportunity to others. "Creative Healing" is her way of giving back, of using her experiences to help others find their path to healing, just as she did.

Through "Creative Healing," Anna not only shares her passion for creativity but also fosters a space of healing and hope. It becomes a project that is not just about art and expression but about transformation and empowerment.

Anna starts putting her plan into action. She reaches out to the community center, proposing her idea for the workshops. They are enthusiastic about the concept and offer her a space to conduct them. She then begins the process of organizing the logistics, from setting a schedule to gathering materials.

Her vision for the workshops includes various creative mediums – writing, painting, music – all intended to provide a safe and supportive space for participants to express themselves and start their healing journeys. She draws upon her own experiences, integrating elements that have helped her, such as mindfulness exercises and group discussions.

To promote her workshops, Anna taps into the network she has built at the bookstore and the support group. She creates flyers and uses social media, generating interest in the local community. The response is positive, with several people signing up, intrigued by the idea of using creativity as a means of healing.

The chapter culminates with the first "Creative Healing" workshop. Anna feels a mix of nerves and excitement as she welcomes a diverse group of participants. The session begins with an introduction, where Anna shares her story, setting a tone of openness and empathy.

As the workshop progresses, the participants engage in various creative activities. Anna guides them gently, offering encouragement and support. She watches as the participants express themselves, some finding solace in painting, others in writing. The atmosphere is one of mutual support and understanding, exactly what Anna had hoped to create.

As Anna reflects on the success of the first workshop. She feels a deep sense of fulfillment, seeing the impact of her initiative on the participants. This project, born from her own experiences, has not only allowed her to give back but has also marked her evolution from someone who once sought support to someone who now provides it.

Anna realizes that this new role of guiding and supporting others is a significant step in her journey, one that adds another layer of meaning to her life. She goes to bed that night with a heart full of gratitude and the knowledge that she is making a difference, turning her past challenges into a source of strength for both herself and her community.

Reflection and Looking Ahead

As the evening settles in, Anna finds herself in her favorite spot by the window, a place that has become her sanctuary for reflection. The room is softly lit, casting a warm and comforting glow. Outside, the city lights twinkle against the night sky, mirroring the quiet flicker of thoughts in Anna's mind.

In this tranquil space, Anna allows herself to truly absorb and reflect on the myriad changes that have colored her life in recent times. She thinks about the challenges she's faced, the fears she's conquered, and the new paths she's bravely traversed.

Anna contemplates the growth that each experience has fostered within her. She reflects on her initial struggles with her past, the journey towards healing, her development into a confident and capable professional, and her deepening bond with Lily. She thinks about her foray into the world of romance again and the fulfillment she's found in giving back to her community through her workshops.

Each of these experiences, Anna realizes, has been like a thread in the tapestry of her life. Some threads have been dark, representing challenges and sorrows, while others have been bright, symbolizing joy and achievements. Together, they form a rich and intricate design, a representation of her life's journey.

Anna acknowledges that the road ahead will undoubtedly hold more challenges. But the sense of trepidation that once would have accompanied this acknowledgment is now replaced by a quiet confidence. She feels equipped with the tools, the support, and the self-awareness to navigate whatever comes her way.

She thinks about her future with a sense of hope and curiosity. Her goals are clearer, her passions rekindled, and her place in the world more firmly established. The possibilities that lie ahead excite her – whether in her career, her personal life, or her continued role in the community.

As Anna journals her reflections, capturing this moment of introspection. She writes not just about where she's been, but also about where she's heading – a future that she looks forward to with optimism and open-heartedness.

As she turns off the light and heads to bed, Anna feels a profound sense of peace. She's grateful for the journey she's on, for the person she's becoming, and for the tapestry of life she's weaving – each thread a valuable part of the whole. She falls asleep with a heart full of gratitude, ready to embrace the new horizons that await her.

Chapter 7:

"Woven Paths"

Mr. Thompson calls a staff meeting to announce the implementation of a new, sophisticated technology system for inventory management. He explains that this change is crucial for the bookstore's efficiency and competitiveness. As he speaks, Anna's mind races with both the potential benefits and the challenges this new system could bring.

Recognizing Anna's proven ability and her recent successes in the managerial role, Mr. Thompson entrusts her with overseeing the implementation of the new system. Anna feels a flutter of anxiety at this significant responsibility but also a sense of pride and determination.

Initially, the technical aspects of the new system seem daunting to Anna. The software is complex, and the transition from the old system promises to be a significant undertaking. But Anna, armed with her resilience and problem-solving skills, dives into the challenge headfirst.

She starts by dedicating time to thoroughly understand the software. Anna arranges for extra training sessions for herself, spending evenings poring over manuals and tutorial videos. Her dedication to mastering the new system is fueled by her commitment to her role and her desire to lead her team effectively through this transition.

As Anna becomes more familiar with the software, she begins to envision innovative ways it could be integrated into the bookstore's existing processes. She suggests enhancements such as linking the inventory system directly to the bookstore's online catalog, streamlining the process for updating online stock levels in real-time.

She also proposes using the system's data analytics capabilities to better understand customer preferences and trends, which could inform future book selections and marketing strategies.

Aware that this change will affect the entire staff, Anna takes a proactive approach to involve her team. She organizes training sessions, ensuring that everyone feels comfortable and competent with the new system. Anna's open and inclusive approach helps to alleviate concerns and fosters a sense of teamwork and shared purpose.

Anna stands in the bookstore after hours, looking over the now-quiet shelves. She reflects on the initial overwhelming feeling when the challenge was first presented and how, through resilience and a willingness to learn, she has turned it into an opportunity for growth – both for herself and the bookstore.

She realizes that every new challenge is a chance to expand her capabilities, echoing the continuous journey of growth and adaptation she has embarked on. With a sense of accomplishment and anticipation for the future, Anna locks up the store, ready for whatever the next day brings.

Deepening Bonds with Lily and Michael

As Anna navigates the complexities of her new role at work, she remains committed to her most important role – being a mother to Lily. To maintain and strengthen their bond, Anna proposes a unique activity: a mother-daughter book club. Lily, with her burgeoning love for reading, is immediately enthused by the idea.

They set aside time each week, creating a cozy nook in their living room with cushions and blankets, surrounded by stacks of books they've chosen together. Each session of their book club involves reading passages aloud, discussing the characters, and sharing their interpretations of the story. It's a time for laughter, learning, and heartfelt conversations.

These book club meetings become a cherished ritual for both Anna and Lily. For Anna, it's not just about fostering Lily's interest in reading but also about connecting with her on a deeper level, understanding her thoughts, fears, and dreams through the stories they share.

Parallel to her time with Lily, Anna's relationship with Michael gradually deepens. They find comfort and joy in each other's company, sharing long walks, engaging conversations, and quiet dinners. Michael shows a genuine interest in Anna's life, respecting her independence and supporting her ambitions.

As Anna manages the challenges of her professional life, Michael becomes a pillar of support. He's understanding when work demands her time, offering help in small but significant ways, like bringing dinner over when she has to work late or suggesting quiet evenings in when she needs to unwind.

Their relationship progresses naturally, with Anna carefully balancing her personal growth and her role as a mother with the budding romance. Michael's presence in her life brings a new dimension of happiness and companionship, something Anna hadn't anticipated but now cherishes.

As Anna reflects on the balancing act of her life. She's a manager, a mother, a partner, and still very much on her journey of personal growth. It's a juggling act that requires patience, time management, and self-care. Anna is mindful to not lose herself in these roles, setting aside time for her own interests and relaxation, ensuring she maintains her sense of self.

Anna sits in her living room, the remnants of the latest book club meeting with Lily around her, and a text from Michael on her phone, planning their next date. She smiles, feeling grateful for the rich tapestry of her life – the challenges, the love, and the growth. It's a delicate balance, but one that she navigates with grace and resilience, embracing each aspect of her life with open arms and an open heart.

Unexpected Reunion

As Anna prepares for her high school reunion, she experiences a complex mix of emotions. Standing before her mirror, she sees not just her reflection but also the echoes of her younger self, a version of her that walked the halls of her high school, unaware of the challenges and triumphs that lay ahead.

Feelings About the Reunion:

1. **Nostalgia and Reflection:** Anna feels a sense of nostalgia as she thinks back to her high school years. It's a bittersweet reminiscence,

acknowledging both the carefree moments and the insecurities of adolescence.

2. **Anxiety:** There's an undercurrent of anxiety about revisiting a past that feels like a lifetime ago. High school reunions often bring back memories and emotions, and for Anna, who has undergone significant changes, the thought of facing old classmates is daunting.

3. **Pride in Her Growth:** Despite the apprehension, Anna also feels a sense of pride. She has grown immensely since those high school days, having faced and overcome personal challenges. The reunion is an opportunity to celebrate her journey and the person she has become.

4. **Curiosity:** There's also a natural curiosity about how her peers have changed and what paths they have taken in life. High school reunions are a chance to reconnect and see the diverse directions everyone's lives have taken.

Bringing Michael as Her Date: As for bringing Michael as her date, Anna deliberates this decision. On one hand, introducing him to her high school peers would be a significant step in their relationship, signaling a level of seriousness and inclusion. Michael, with his understanding and supportive nature, could be a comforting presence for her.

On the other hand, Anna is conscious of the fact that their relationship is still relatively new. She values the independence she's worked hard to achieve and may choose to navigate the reunion on her own terms, without the dynamics of a date. Additionally, Anna may want to focus on her own experiences and connections at the reunion without the added dimension of managing a partner's introduction to her past life.

Ultimately, Anna's decision, whether to bring Michael or attend solo, would reflect her comfort level and the pace at which she wishes to take her relationship. If she decides to bring him, it could be a meaningful step in their growing relationship. If she chooses to go alone, it's a testament to her self-reliance and confidence in facing her past independently. Either way, the reunion stands as a significant evening for Anna, a moment to acknowledge her past, embrace her present, and look forward to her future.

Anna finds herself preparing for an event she has mixed feelings about – her high school reunion. The invitation evokes a flood of memories, some pleasant, others less so. High school had been a time of self-discovery but also of insecurities and challenges.

On the evening of the reunion, Anna stands before her mirror, reflecting on the person she was back then and the woman she has become. She takes a deep breath, steadying her nerves, and decides to face the evening as an opportunity to celebrate her growth rather than dread confronting her past.

The reunion is held in the high school gymnasium, transformed with decorations that evoke a sense of nostalgia. As Anna steps in, she's greeted by familiar faces, some of whom she hasn't seen since graduation. The initial interactions are a whirlwind of introductions and shared memories.

Among the crowd, Anna encounters people who remind her of both good and challenging times. She meets old friends with whom she reconnects effortlessly, reminiscing about their youthful adventures. But there are also encounters that test her – former classmates who had once been part of her struggles, either directly or indirectly.

One encounter stands out when Anna comes face-to-face with a former classmate who had been unkind to her in their teenage years. The encounter initially sends a ripple of discomfort through her, but she quickly composes herself. Anna engages in conversation with a calm and polite demeanor, showcasing her maturity and the confidence she has cultivated.

During her high school years, Anna experienced unkindness from a particular classmate, a memory that remains vivid in her mind. This classmate, let's call her Rachel, was part of a popular group in school and often exhibited behaviors that were hurtful to others, including Anna.

Nature of Unkindness:

1. **Verbal Bullying:** Rachel frequently made disparaging remarks about Anna, often in front of others. These comments could range from mocking Anna's appearance to belittling her academic achievements or interests. This verbal bullying left Anna feeling self-conscious and diminished her sense of self-worth during those formative years.
2. **Social Exclusion:** Rachel often orchestrated social exclusion tactics, deliberately leaving Anna out of group activities or gatherings. This exclusion was not only painful in the moment but also contributed to a lasting sense of loneliness and isolation for Anna during her high school years.
3. **Rumors and Gossip:** Rachel was known to spread rumors or gossip about Anna, which not only affected Anna's social life but also added to her anxiety and stress. These rumors often painted Anna in a negative light, based on falsehoods or exaggerations.

Coming face-to-face with Rachel at the reunion initially sends a jolt of discomfort through Anna, as old memories resurface. However, Anna's response to this encounter is a testament to the tremendous personal growth she has experienced since her high school days. She composes herself quickly, refusing to revert to the hurt and insecurity she once felt.

Engaging in conversation with Rachel, Anna demonstrates a calm and polite demeanor. She converses with a maturity and confidence that is worlds apart from the teenager Rachel once knew. This poise is not about showing superiority or seeking validation; rather, it is Anna's way of acknowledging her past without letting it define her.

This interaction is significant for Anna. It's a moment where she confronts a painful part of her past, not with bitterness or anger, but with grace and composure. It highlights how far she has come in her journey of self-acceptance and empowerment. By handling the situation with such dignity, Anna closes a chapter on her old insecurities and reaffirms the strong, self-assured person she has become.

This interaction becomes a significant moment for Anna. She realizes that the opinions and actions of others in her past no longer define her. She has moved beyond the insecurities of her teenage years, embracing her journey and the person she has become.

As the evening winds down, Anna finds a quiet corner to gather her thoughts. The reunion, with all its mixed emotions, serves as a poignant reminder of her journey. She acknowledges the impact her past has had on shaping her, but also recognizes that she is no longer the same person who walked the halls of her high school.

Anna leaves the reunion with a sense of closure and a renewed appreciation for her journey. The experience reinforces her understanding that while the past is a part of who she is, it does not dictate her future. She drives home feeling a sense of peace, grateful for the experiences that have led her to this point in her life and excited for what lies ahead.

Following the uplifting experience at her high school reunion, Anna channels her renewed energy into further developing her "Creative Healing" workshops. The initial series, which focused primarily on visual arts as a means of expression and healing, had been well-received, sparking a desire in Anna to broaden its scope.

She begins by reaching out to local artists and therapists, building a network of professionals who share her vision of using creative outlets for emotional and mental well-being. Her idea is to create a more holistic program that incorporates various forms of artistic expression.

Anna's efforts lead to fruitful collaborations. She meets with a music therapist who introduces the idea of integrating music therapy sessions into the workshops. They plan activities where participants can explore their emotions through music, whether by listening, playing instruments, or even composing.

Additionally, Anna connects with a local writer and creative writing instructor. Together, they develop a module for the workshops focused on writing as therapy. This includes journaling, poetry, and storytelling, offering participants new ways to articulate their feelings and experiences.

With these collaborations in place, Anna launches the expanded version of her "Creative Healing" workshops. The program now boasts a diverse range of activities, catering to different interests and forms of expression.

The response from the community is overwhelmingly positive. More people begin to participate, drawn by the variety of the sessions and the welcoming, inclusive atmosphere that Anna and her team foster. Participants range from those dealing with personal traumas to individuals simply seeking a creative outlet for stress relief.

As the workshops progress, Anna witnesses the transformative power of creative expression. She sees participants who had initially been reserved slowly open, finding their voice through their chosen medium. Whether it's through a painted canvas, a melody, or a written piece, each person finds a unique way to express and heal.

Anna Again reflects on the impact of the "Creative Healing" workshops. She realizes that what started as a small initiative based on her personal journey has grown into a valuable community resource. She feels a deep sense of fulfillment, knowing that she's not only found healing for herself but is also facilitating it for others.

In her journal, Anna writes about this expansion of her project, noting how it parallels her own growth. She acknowledges the challenges ahead in managing this growing initiative but feels equipped and inspired to continue this work.

Personal Reflection and Growth

As the narrative of Anna's life unfolds, she recognizes the need for a pause, a moment to reconnect with herself amidst her bustling life. She decides to attend a weekend retreat at a serene location nestled in nature, a place where she can immerse herself in tranquility and self-care.

The retreat that Anna attends is nestled in a tranquil and picturesque setting, an idyllic haven far removed from the hustle and bustle of city life. The location is a serene landscape, where verdant forests meet meandering streams, creating an atmosphere that is both calming and rejuvenating. It's an environment that encourages introspection and offers a much-needed escape for relaxation and self-discovery.

Retreat Features and Activities:

1. **Natural Beauty:** The retreat is set in a location that boasts natural beauty. Tall, majestic trees surround the area, offering ample shade and a sense of being close to nature. The gentle sounds of flowing water from nearby streams add a soothing background melody, enhancing the peaceful ambiance of the setting.
2. **Guided Meditation Sessions:** A key feature of the retreat's program is the guided meditation sessions. These sessions are led by experienced instructors who help participants explore various meditation techniques, focusing on mindfulness and deep relaxation. The sessions are designed to suit both beginners and those more experienced with meditation, making them accessible and beneficial for everyone.
3. **Nature Walks:** The retreat includes guided nature walks, allowing participants to immerse themselves in the surrounding beauty. These walks are not just physical activities but also opportunities for mindful observation and connection with the environment. Participants

are encouraged to take in the sights, sounds, and smells of nature, fostering a deeper appreciation of the natural world.

4. **Mindfulness Workshops:** The retreat offers workshops focused on mindfulness and self-awareness. These workshops cover topics such as managing stress, cultivating positive thinking, and developing emotional resilience. They provide practical tools and techniques that participants can apply in their daily lives.

5. **Self-Reflection Opportunities:** The retreat's schedule also allows for periods of personal time for self-reflection. Participants can use these moments to journal, meditate privately, or simply enjoy the tranquility of the surroundings.

6. **Community and Connection:** While much of the retreat is focused on personal growth, there is also an emphasis on building a sense of community among participants. Shared meals, group activities, and open discussions create a supportive and inclusive environment.

7. **Accommodation and Amenities:** The retreat offers comfortable accommodations that blend in with the natural surroundings. The rooms are designed to provide a restful and contemplative space, free from the distractions of everyday life. Healthy, nourishing meals are provided, often featuring local and organic ingredients.

For Anna, this retreat represents an opportunity to step back from her daily responsibilities and focus on her own well-being. It's a chance to deepen her practice of mindfulness, connect with nature, and gain new insights into her personal growth journey. The combination of the serene setting, expert-led sessions, and the supportive community creates an enriching experience that has the potential to impact her long after the retreat concludes.

On her first morning at the retreat, Anna joins a group for a nature walk. As they wander through the lush greenery, the guide encourages them to observe the environment mindfully, to listen to the rustling leaves, the chirping birds, and to feel the texture of the earth beneath their feet. This exercise in mindfulness helps Anna to be fully present, allowing her to momentarily set aside her usual concerns and immerse herself in the peacefulness of nature.

The meditation sessions become a profound experience for Anna. Seated in a quiet room, with soft natural light filtering in, she learns techniques to quiet her mind and focus on her breathing. These moments of stillness bring clarity and calm, helping her to delve deeper into her thoughts and emotions.

During these sessions, Anna confronts feelings and thoughts she has been too busy to address – her fears about her new responsibilities, her hopes for her relationship with Michael, and her aspirations for the future. She faces these thoughts with honesty and openness, allowing herself to process and understand them.

In the evenings, Anna spends time journaling in her room, which overlooks a serene garden. This practice becomes a key part of her retreat experience. She writes about her reflections from the day, her feelings during the meditation sessions, and her thoughts during the nature walks.

Journaling provides her with a means to articulate her internal journey, capturing her insights, revelations, and the areas of her life she still wishes to work on. She writes about balancing her roles as a mother, a professional, and a partner, and how this retreat is helping her to find harmony within this balance.

As the retreat comes to an end, Anna feels rejuvenated and more connected with herself. She has gained new perspectives on her life's path, feeling a sense of renewal in her commitment to her personal and professional goals.

with Anna driving back home, her mind and spirit refreshed. She feels ready to return to her daily life, armed with new tools and insights to maintain her inner peace amidst the busyness of her world.

A New Opportunity

Upon returning from her retreat, rejuvenated and filled with new insights, Anna receives an intriguing proposal. A local community college, having heard of the success of her "Creative Healing" workshops, reaches out to her with an offer to teach a course on creative arts as a form of therapy.

The course would be part of the college's continuing education program, aimed at individuals interested in exploring creative methods for personal development and healing. The college believes Anna's unique blend of personal experience and practical application in her workshops makes her the ideal candidate to lead this course.

Anna is both excited and apprehensive about this new opportunity. The prospect of sharing her knowledge and techniques with a wider audience, and potentially impacting more lives, aligns perfectly with her passion. She envisions a classroom where she can guide students in discovering the therapeutic power of creativity, much like she has.

However, Anna is also aware of the demands this new role would place on her time and energy. Balancing her managerial duties at the bookstore, her responsibilities as a mother, her relationship with Michael, and now the potential of a teaching position poses a significant challenge.

To aid her decision-making, Anna turns to her support network. She discusses the opportunity with Mr. Thompson, who encourages her to pursue it, offering flexibility in her bookstore schedule. She talks it over with Michael, who is supportive and reassures her of his willingness to help where he can, especially in balancing her time.

Most importantly, Anna sits down with Lily to explain the opportunity and what it might mean for their time together. Lily, wise beyond her years, encourages her mother to take the chance, expressing pride in Anna's abilities and achievements.

After much thought and discussion, Anna decides to accept the offer. She sees this as not just a professional opportunity but as a step forward in her journey – a chance to expand her impact and explore a new facet of her passion for creative arts therapy.

Anna prepares her curriculum for the course, feeling a blend of nervousness and excitement. She realizes that this new role is a testament to her journey – from seeking healing to providing it. It's a moment that underscores her growth, resilience, and her commitment to spreading the message of healing through creativity.

Anna looks out of her window, reflecting on the intertwining paths her life has taken. Each decision, each step she has taken, has led her to this moment – a moment where she stands not only as a learner but also as a teacher, ready to embark on this new chapter of her life.

Making a Choice

Anna has carefully considered the teaching opportunity, knowing it could open new avenues in her life. However, she is also acutely aware of the need to maintain balance in her various roles.

In seeking counsel, Anna first turns to Lily. They sit together in their cozy living room, surrounded by the many books they've shared. Anna explains what the teaching role entails and how it might affect their time together. Lily, showing maturity beyond her years, listens intently. She asks thoughtful questions, showing an understanding of her mother's passions and aspirations. Ultimately, Lily encourages Anna, expressing her support and pride in her mother's achievements.

Later, Anna discusses the opportunity with Michael over a quiet dinner. Michael listens, his eyes reflecting his deep understanding of Anna's aspirations and his unwavering support for her. He encourages her to seize the opportunity, reassuring her of his willingness to be there for her, to help navigate the complexities of balancing this new role with her personal life.

Alone later that evening, Anna reflects on the conversations with Lily and Michael, and on her own desires and ambitions. She recognizes that teaching this course not only aligns with her professional goals but also resonates with her personal journey of healing and growth. It represents a chance to share her knowledge, to inspire others, and to continue her own path of self-discovery and development.

With clarity and a sense of purpose, Anna decides to accept the teaching position. She feels a mix of excitement and responsibility as she drafts an email to the community college, confirming her acceptance.

Anna sitting back in her chair, a feeling of contentment washing over her. She realizes that each step she has taken, each decision she has made, has been part of a larger journey – one that has led her to this point of embracing new challenges and opportunities.

Anna reflects on how her life is a tapestry of experiences, each thread woven with its own story, its own lessons. She acknowledges that the path ahead may have its uncertainties, but she feels equipped and eager to meet them.

As she turns off the light and heads to bed, Anna feels grateful for the love and support of Lily and Michael, and for the journey that has brought her to this moment. She falls asleep with a heart full of hope, ready to embark on this new chapter of her life, confident in her ability to weave these new experiences into the rich tapestry of her ever-evolving story.

Anna in a reflective state, gazing out her window into the tranquil night. The stars twinkle in the vast expanse above, mirroring the multitude of possibilities and paths that lay before her. In this quiet moment, she allows herself to fully absorb the sense of accomplishment and the vibrant anticipation for the future that she feels.

Anna reflects on the journey that has brought her to this point. She thinks about the challenges she's faced, the obstacles she's overcome, and the victories she's celebrated. Each experience has been a thread in the intricate tapestry of her life, weaving a story of resilience, growth, and transformation.

She remembers the times of doubt and uncertainty, how they had once seemed insurmountable. Yet, here she is, having navigated through them with strength she hadn't known she possessed. This realization fills her with a profound sense of empowerment.

Her thoughts then turn to the wider impact of her actions. Through her "Creative Healing" workshops and now the upcoming teaching role, Anna is extending her influence beyond her personal sphere. She is contributing something meaningful to her community, using her experiences and insights to foster growth and healing in others. This role of being a giver, a nurturer, and an inspirer is something she cherishes deeply.

Looking forward, Anna feels a thrilling blend of excitement and curiosity. Her life is no longer a series of reactions to circumstances but a proactive journey of choices and opportunities. She envisions her future – teaching, continuing her work at the bookstore, nurturing her relationship with Lily and Michael, and perhaps exploring new avenues in her personal and professional life.

Anna jotting down a few thoughts in her journal, a habit that has become her anchor and her compass. She writes about her gratitude, her hopes, and her dreams. She pens down a promise to herself to continue embracing each new day with openness and courage.

As she turns off the light and settles into bed, Anna feels a comforting sense of peace. Her path, woven with diverse experiences, is uniquely hers – rich in learning, filled with love, and brimming with the promise of new beginnings. She drifts off to sleep, not just dreaming of the future but actively looking forward to crafting it with her own hands.

Chapter 8:

"Charting New Courses"

The morning sun streams through the windows of the classroom, casting a warm glow on the rows of desks. Anna stands at the front of the room, her heart fluttering with a blend of nervousness and excitement. It's her first day as an instructor for the creative arts therapy course, a moment that marks a significant milestone in her journey.

The students begin to file in, each carrying their own stories and reasons for being there. Anna greets them with a welcoming smile, trying to ease the palpable anticipation in the room. She arranges her notes on the podium, her hands slightly trembling, but her spirit buoyed by the passion for what she is about to do.

As the class settles, Anna takes a deep breath and begins her lecture. She introduces herself, not just as an instructor but as someone who has personally experienced the transformative power of creative arts in healing and self-discovery. She shares snippets of her journey, from the challenges she faced to the coping mechanisms she found in creative expression.

Anna's openness sets a tone of trust and authenticity in the classroom. Her anecdotes about using painting and writing as tools for emotional exploration and expression captivate the students. They listen, some nodding in understanding, others visibly moved by the honesty in her words.

As Anna stands at the front of the classroom, her presence is one of calm assurance mixed with genuine openness. The atmosphere in the room is one of attentive anticipation as the students, a diverse group with varying experiences and backgrounds, prepare to embark on a journey of creative exploration under Anna's guidance.

Anna begins by sharing her personal experiences with painting and writing. Her stories are not just narratives; they are vivid, emotive expressions of her journey. She talks about how a blank canvas, or an empty page can serve as a safe space for unfiltered expression, a place to channel emotions, fears, hopes, and dreams.

Her anecdotes are deeply relatable. She speaks of moments when words failed her, and how colors and brushstrokes became her voice. She recalls times when writing in her journal helped her untangle the complex web of her thoughts and emotions. These stories resonate with the students, some of whom have experienced similar struggles with expressing themselves.

Anna's honesty about her challenges, including her past traumas and the path to healing, strikes a chord. Her willingness to be vulnerable in front of the class sets a tone of trust and authenticity. It encourages a similar openness among the students, fostering an environment where vulnerability is not seen as a weakness but as a courageous step towards self-awareness and healing.

As Anna continues to speak in the classroom, her words seem to resonate on a deeper level with the students, creating an atmosphere charged with empathy and introspection. The room, typically a space for academic learning, transforms into a haven for emotional exploration and connection.

The students are visibly engaged, leaning forward in their seats, hanging onto Anna's every word. As she shares her experiences with painting and writing, how these forms of creative expression helped her navigate through her darkest times and celebrate her brightest moments, there's a palpable sense of empathy in the room. Her honesty and vulnerability act as a bridge, connecting her with the students on a deeply human level.

reflections on the exercises. A sense of camaraderie begins to develop among them, fostered by the safe and open environment Anna has created.

By the end of the session, Anna's initial nervousness has transformed into a sense of fulfillment. She looks around at the students, now animatedly discussing the day's activities, and feels a deep sense of satisfaction. She has not only imparted knowledge but has also sparked a flame of curiosity and self-exploration in her students.

Anna collects her materials after the students have left, the echoes of their discussions still lingering in the air. She feels a profound connection to her new role – it's not just about teaching; it's about guiding and inspiring others on their paths to healing. As she locks the classroom door behind her, she's filled with a sense of purpose and anticipation for the rest of the semester.

The Bookstore's New Chapter

Back at the bookstore, Anna's creative energy is in full swing. She's in the midst of organizing a series of author events and book signings, an initiative that has breathed new life into the store. Local and regional authors are invited to speak, their sessions ranging from readings to engaging discussions about their writing processes and the themes of their works.

These events transform the bookstore into a vibrant community hub, attracting book lovers of all ages. The store buzzes with excitement on event days, filled with the anticipation of meeting authors and the joy of discovering new stories.

Anna's efforts pay off significantly. Each event draws a sizable crowd, leading to increased sales and heightened customer engagement. The bookstore's social media pages, managed by Anna with a blend of personal touch and professional flair, come alive with updates and photos from the events, further amplifying interest and reach.

The local community starts to recognize the bookstore not just as a retail space but as a cultural center, a place where literature comes alive and readers can connect with authors and each other.

Impressed with the renewed energy and success of the bookstore under Anna's management, Mr. Thompson calls her for a meeting to discuss the future. He commends her for her innovative approach and shares his thoughts about expanding the bookstore's presence into the online realm.

Anna listens, her mind already brimming with ideas. She envisions an online store that offers more than just books – a platform for virtual author events, a blog featuring book reviews and literary discussions, and perhaps an online book club.

Embracing this new challenge, Anna begins to strategize the bookstore's digital expansion. She considers partnering with local web designers and digital marketing professionals to create an engaging and user-friendly online platform.

She also proposes interactive features for the website, such as a section where customers can share their book reviews, a monthly newsletter featuring staff picks and upcoming events, and an online forum for readers to discuss their favorite books.

Anna is seen outlining a proposal for the bookstore's online expansion. Her desk is scattered with notes and sketches of the website layout, a testament to her thorough and creative planning process.

While Anna looks out the bookstore window, contemplating the journey ahead. She feels a surge of excitement at the prospect of bringing the charm and community spirit of the bookstore into the digital world. Anna's growth is evident – from managing the store's day-to-day operations to spearheading its expansion into new territories. Her journey continues to be one of innovation, leadership, and unwavering commitment to her passions.

Lily's Growing Independence

As Anna immerses herself in her professional projects, she simultaneously navigates a poignant shift in her personal life. Lily, now a teenager, is stepping into a phase of increased independence and self-discovery. This transition is bittersweet for Anna, who feels a mixture of pride in Lily's growth and a wistful nostalgia for the days when Lily was younger.

Anna observes subtle changes in Lily – the way she begins to assert her opinions more confidently, her burgeoning interests that stretch beyond the family sphere, and her desire for more autonomy. While Anna encourages this independence, she also grapples with the emotional complexity of letting go and allowing Lily to make her own decisions and mistakes.

Their mother-daughter book club, a cherished tradition, continues but undergoes its own transformation. The books they choose become more sophisticated, delving into complex themes and characters. Their discussions during these book club sessions grow deeper, often veering into philosophical territories and reflecting Lily's developing intellect and worldview.

These book club meetings become a space where Lily freely expresses her thoughts and feelings, not just about the books but also about her life – her aspirations, her challenges at school, and her perspectives on various issues. Anna listens, often

Attending concerts and musical events is another avenue through which they deepen their relationship. Whether it's a classical music performance at a grand concert hall, a jazz night at a local club, or an outdoor music festival, these experiences allow them to appreciate the power and beauty of live music together. The shared experience of listening, feeling the music, and being part of an audience adds a communal dimension to their enjoyment.

Exploring the local theater scene offers them both entertainment and a glimpse into diverse narratives and storytelling styles. Whether it's a well-known Broadway show, an experimental play by an emerging playwright, or a community theater production, each experience is a journey into different worlds and perspectives. Discussions often follow these outings, where they exchange views on the storyline, the performances, and the production's overall impact.

These cultural outings are not just about indulging in known interests but also about discovering new ones. Anna might introduce Michael to an art genre he's unfamiliar with, or Michael might suggest a musical style Anna hasn't explored before. This openness to new experiences keeps their outings exciting and enriching.

These outings serve as a platform for Anna and Michael to connect over shared interests and appreciate each other's insights and perspectives. They offer a break from the routine of daily life, creating special moments and memories. Moreover, these experiences provide intellectual stimulation and emotional resonance, contributing to the depth and richness of their relationship.

Through these cultural outings, Anna and Michael's relationship grows in a shared space of appreciation for arts and culture. These experiences not only bring joy but also strengthen their bond, adding layers of understanding, enjoyment, and mutual respect.

Quiet evenings at home become a cherished part of their relationship. Sometimes, these evenings involve cooking together, with the kitchen filled with laughter and the aromas of shared meals. Other times, they're content to simply sit together, perhaps reading in companionable silence or sharing thoughts and reflections on their day.

On some evenings, the kitchen becomes a lively space of collaboration and creativity. Cooking together turns into an enjoyable activity, far beyond the routine of meal preparation. They pick out recipes to try, sometimes challenging themselves with new cuisines or indulging in comfort foods. As they cook, the kitchen is filled with the sounds of sizzling, chopping, and the occasional clink of wine glasses. Laughter often accompanies their culinary experiments, whether they're celebrating a successful dish or salvaging a not-so-perfect one. These moments in the kitchen become about more than just food; they're an expression of their partnership and enjoyment of life's everyday joys.

Other evenings are more subdued. Anna and Michael might find contentment in sitting together quietly, each with a book in hand. This companionable silence is a testament to their comfort with each other, finding peace in simply being in the same space. Occasionally, one would share a snippet from their book or a thought it sparked, leading to a gentle, reflective conversation. These quiet evenings of reading and relaxation offer a pause from the outside world, a time to recharge and connect in the simplest way.

Sometimes, their evenings at home are spent sharing thoughts and reflections on their day. These conversations can range from casual talks about daily events to deeper discussions about their dreams, fears, and aspirations. These discussions are a way for Anna and Michael to maintain an emotional connection, understanding and supporting each other through life's ups and downs.

These quiet evenings at home gradually weave into the fabric of their relationship, creating a shared space that is both comforting and nurturing. It's a space where they can be themselves, where the pace of life slows down, and where they can appreciate the simple, yet profound, aspects of their connection.

For Anna, these evenings are a significant shift from her past experiences. They represent a balance of independence and togetherness, a harmonious blend of personal space and shared intimacy. For both Anna and Michael, these moments are an essential part of building a relationship that is grounded in mutual respect, understanding, and a deep appreciation of the joys of everyday life.

During these intimate moments, Anna and Michael engage in deep conversations, discussing everything from personal philosophies to future dreams. Michael listens with a kind of attentiveness that makes Anna feel truly heard and understood. He shares his own experiences and insights, offering perspectives that challenge and inspire Anna.

Occasionally, Anna and Michael take trips to explore new places. Whether it's a weekend getaway to a nearby town or a day spent hiking in nature, these excursions add an element of adventure to their relationship. These experiences bring them closer, as they navigate new environments and create shared memories.

On one such trip, as they walk along a scenic trail, Anna realizes how much Michael has come to mean to her. He is more than just a romantic partner; he is a confidant, a supporter, and a source of strength. His presence in her life has brought a sense of completeness and joy that she hadn't known was missing.

During a weekend getaway, Anna and Michael find themselves on a scenic trail, immersed in the natural beauty of a lush landscape. The trail winds through a verdant forest, with sunlight filtering through the canopy of leaves, casting dappled shadows on their path. The air is fresh and invigorating, filled with the sounds of birds and the gentle rustle of leaves. It's an idyllic setting that seems to heighten the sense of connection and tranquility between them.

As they walk, sometimes in conversation and sometimes in comfortable silence, Anna becomes acutely aware of the profound impact Michael has had on her life. It's a realization that blooms quietly but unmistakably in her heart. Michael, with his understanding nature and steady presence, has grown to be much more than a romantic partner. He's become a pillar in her life – a confidant whom she can trust with her deepest thoughts and fears, a supporter who encourages her dreams and aspirations, and a source of strength that complements her own resilience.

Anna notices the little things that encapsulate his importance in her life – the way he listens attentively, showing genuine interest in her words; how he shares his own thoughts and vulnerabilities, creating a mutual space of trust and openness; his ability to make her laugh even in moments of doubt, bringing lightness to her life. His presence has become a comforting and stabilizing force, offering a balance of love, support, and companionship.

This realization brings with it a sense of completeness and joy. Anna understands that Michael has filled a space in her life she hadn't fully recognized was there. It's not that he completes her – she is whole on her own – but rather that his presence enriches her life in ways she hadn't anticipated. With him, she experiences a sense of partnership that is nurturing and fulfilling.

As they continue their walk, with the beauty of nature surrounding them, Anna finds herself reflecting on the journey that has brought her to this moment. From the challenges of her past to the growth and healing she has undergone, every step has led her to this feeling of contentment and happiness. In Michael, she has found not just love, but a true partner in the fullest sense – someone who stands by her as they both navigate the path of life together.

Anna and Michael sitting on a park bench, watching the sunset. They talk about their future, not making concrete plans, but sharing a mutual understanding that they want to continue this journey together.

As they sit there, Anna reflects on the serendipity of their meeting and how their relationship has grown. She appreciates the balance Michael brings to her life – the way he supports her ambitions while also providing a space for relaxation and joy. She feels grateful for his presence in her life, recognizing the strength and stability that their relationship offers.

A New Community Project

Buoyed by the positive impact of her teaching and her innovations at the bookstore, Anna is inspired to take her passion for creativity and community engagement a step further. She conceives the idea of a literary and arts festival, a community event that would celebrate the diverse talents of local artists and writers while fostering a sense of community.

Anna envisions a festival that is more than just a showcase of creativity; she sees it as a platform for dialogue, learning, and connection. It would feature book readings, art exhibitions, workshops, and panel discussions, all aimed at bringing people together and highlighting the importance of art in community building.

Anna begins reaching out to various local artists, writers, and business owners, sharing her vision for the festival. She finds that her enthusiasm is contagious, and soon she has a collaborative team, each member bringing their unique skills and ideas to the table.

They hold planning meetings in the bookstore after hours, the space brimming with energy and creativity. Discussions revolve around themes for the festival, potential participants, and logistical considerations. Local businesses offer sponsorships and venues for events, excited to be part of something that promises to enliven the community.

As word of the festival spreads, the community's excitement grows. Anna and her team create a buzz using social media, local media, and word-of-mouth. They organize a series of pre-festival events – like pop-up art installations and mini-readings in public spaces – to build anticipation and engage the community.

Volunteers from the community come forward to help, drawn by the festival's inclusive and celebratory spirit. High school and college students, retired professionals, and local residents all offer their time and skills, creating a sense of shared ownership and pride in the event.

The day of the festival arrives, transforming a local park and several nearby venues into vibrant hubs of artistic expression and cultural exchange. There are tents for book signings, areas for art workshops, stages for readings and performances, and spaces for panel discussions on various literary and artistic topics.

Anna moves through the festival, a blend of organizer, participant, and observer. She watches as people of all ages interact with the artists and authors, engage in workshops, and immerse themselves in the creative atmosphere. The air is filled with the sounds of lively discussions, laughter, and the shared joy of discovery.

As the festival draws to a close, Anna stands on a small stage to thank everyone involved. Looking out at the faces in the crowd – sparkling with inspiration and satisfaction – she feels a deep sense of accomplishment. The festival has not only celebrated creativity but has also woven tighter bonds within the community.

Anna walks through the now-quiet park, post-festival. She reflects on the journey that led her here, from seeking personal healing to fostering a community-wide celebration of creativity. She feels a profound connection to her community and a reinvigorated passion for her work. As she locks up the bookstore that night, her heart is full of gratitude and excitement for the future, eager to see how this new path will unfold in her ever-woven tapestry of life.

Reflecting on Balance and Growth

While Anna is in her garden, a space that has become a sanctuary for her thoughts and reflections. Surrounded by the lush greenery and vibrant blooms that she and Lily have nurtured together, Anna finds a moment of peace amidst her busy life. The garden, with its flourishing life, serves as a metaphor for her own growth and the blossoming of her various endeavors.

As she sits with her journal, the soft evening light casting gentle shadows, Anna contemplates the delicate balance of the roles she plays. She thinks about her days at the college, filled with the enthusiasm and curiosity of her students, and the satisfaction of sharing her knowledge and experiences. She reflects on the bustling energy of the bookstore, where her ideas have brought new life and connected her with a diverse community of book lovers.

Her thoughts then turn to Lily, growing more independent each day, yet still her beacon of love and motivation. She considers her relationship with Michael, a partnership that has brought unexpected joy and support into her life. And she thinks about her role as a community leader, how organizing the festival has linked her more deeply with her surroundings.

In her journal, Anna writes about how each aspect of her life, while distinct, is intricately woven together. Her role as a teacher enriches her perspectives as a bookstore manager; her experiences as a mother provide depth to her relationships and community work; and her personal journey of growth and healing informs her teaching and leadership.

She acknowledges the challenges that come with juggling these roles – the time constraints, the emotional labor, and the constant need for adaptation. Yet, she also recognizes the immense fulfillment each role brings. They are threads of different colors and textures, each contributing to the richness of her life's tapestry.

Anna's journal entry ends with expressions of gratitude and hope. She writes about her gratitude for the journey she has been on, for the people who have supported her, and for the opportunities that have allowed her to grow and contribute. She looks to the future with anticipation, excited for the continuing evolution of her life and the paths yet to be explored.

As Anna closes her journal and gazes out into the twilight of her garden, she feels a profound sense of contentment and purpose. The challenges and rewards of her multifaceted life merge into a harmonious balance. She stands up, takes a deep breath of the fresh evening air, and steps back into the house, ready to embrace whatever comes next with the resilience and openness that have become her hallmarks.

About the Author

Kyleen is a passionate storyteller and advocate for personal growth and resilience. Born and raised in OR, Kyleen has always been drawn to the power of narrative to inspire, heal, and bring people together.

From a young age, Kyleen found solace and joy in both reading and writing. She spent countless hours immersed in books, which ignited a lifelong love for literature and a deep appreciation for the written word. Kyleen pursued her passion, earning a degree in Healthcare Administration.

Before becoming an author, Kyleen worked as a CNA, an experience that enriched her understanding of human nature and the complexities of life. She draws from these experiences in her writing, crafting stories that are not only engaging but also deeply reflective of the human experience.

"Unbroken Harmony: A Journey of Hope and Resilience" is Kyleen's debut novel. Inspired by personal experiences, observations of resilience in others, or a specific event], the book is a testament to her belief in the enduring strength of the human spirit. Through her writing, Kyleen seeks to offer hope, encourage reflection, and celebrate the unyielding resilience that lies within each of us.

When not writing, Kyleen enjoys being with her family, exploring the beauty of all around her.

Kyleen continues to write and is already working on her next project, eager to share more stories that resonate and inspire.